MEDICAL MYTHS THAT CAN KILL YOU

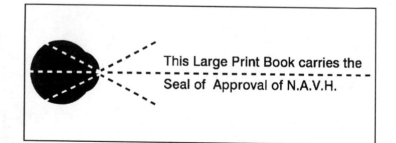

This Large Print Book carries the
Seal of Approval of N.A.V.H.

MEDICAL MYTHS THAT CAN KILL YOU

AND THE 101 TRUTHS THAT WILL SAVE, EXTEND, AND IMPROVE YOUR LIFE

NANCY L. SNYDERMAN, M.D., F.A.C.S.
CHIEF MEDICAL EDITOR, NBC NEWS

THORNDIKE PRESS
A part of Gale, Cengage Learning

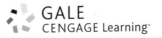
GALE
CENGAGE Learning

Detroit • New York • San Francisco • New Haven, Conn • Waterville, Maine • London

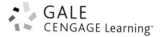

GALE
CENGAGE Learning™

Thorndike Press® Large Print Health, Home & Learning.

The text of this Large Print edition is unabridged.

Other aspects of the book may vary from the original edition.

Set in 16 pt. Plantin.

Printed on permanent paper.

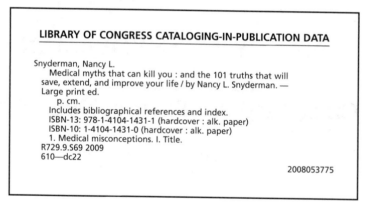

LIBRARY OF CONGRESS CATALOGING-IN-PUBLICATION DATA

Snyderman, Nancy L.
    Medical myths that can kill you : and the 101 truths that will save, extend, and improve your life / by Nancy L. Snyderman. — Large print ed.
        p. cm.
    Includes bibliographical references and index.
    ISBN-13: 978-1-4104-1431-1 (hardcover : alk. paper)
    ISBN-10: 1-4104-1431-0 (hardcover : alk. paper)
    1. Medical misconceptions. I. Title.
R729.9.S69 2009
610—dc22

                                          2008053775

Published in 2009 in arrangement with Crown Publishers, a division of Random House, Inc.

Printed in the United States of America
1 2 3 4 5 6 7 12 11 10 09

To my parents, Joy and Sandy,
who have taught me that good food, good
  exercise, and
good health all go together.

To my children, Kate, Rachel, and Charlie,
who have already learned how to embrace
  life, and
to my husband, Doug,
who always gives me the time and space to
  be me.

ACKNOWLEDGMENTS

It's one thing to conceive an idea. It's quite another to turn it into something, and to do that you need a nucleus of great people around you. Any project is as much about the people who surround you and invest in your thoughts as it is about you. The easiest and worst thing to do is gather folks who are unimaginative, unchallenging, and not invested in the project. In this case, I couldn't have been luckier.

I had a kernel of an idea and had three brilliant women help me take it from there. Working relationships and friendships were forged from New Jersey to San Francisco to New York to Texas, a real cross-country collaboration. Brief meetings, phone conversations, e-mails, and faxes accomplished the technical parts of pulling the book together; friendships and camaraderie cemented the rest.

Amy Rennert and I didn't need a contract

to start working together. She is a woman who speaks from the heart and confirms a deal with a handshake. Ours was a friendship forged instantly. Amy is my agent and friend who "got it" even when I lost sight and meandered. She has been a constant sounding board and advocate every step of the way.

Maggie Greenwood-Robinson was the next part of the equation. Maggie steered, organized, researched, and helped me put my thoughts into cohesive sentences. She kept me honest and on time. She poked and prodded and kept this surgeon-author on track. Her inquisitive mind and passion for challenging the status quo helped me reframe questions from the patient's point of view.

Heather Jackson is an extraordinary editor who immersed herself in every part of this book. She brainstormed, suggested, and challenged the entire team to think and create beyond the obvious. She is passionate about the process, as well as the final product, and is a wonderfully constructive critic. Heather guided us with class and encouragement, showing us on every page how to do it even better.

Two women who would not expect to find themselves acknowledged here are Ami

Schmitz and Kerri Zimmer. Ami was my producer at ABC News and is again my producer at NBC News. We have worked together for fifteen years and counting now. She has the keenest news sense, able to pinpoint what is newsworthy and, just as important, what is not. She continues to keep me honest and always has her eye on the ball. Kerri Zimmer has been invaluable in the preparation of this book, keeping briefing notes from our segments on the *Today* show and tracking down contacts and stray journal articles. These women are trustworthy and smart and make my life as a television journalist great fun.

Andrea Alstrup and I met during my tenure at Johnson & Johnson. As a woman who started her career as an assistant to an assistant and who retired as one of Johnson & Johnson's top executives, she is a stunning example that we can all carve out the lives we dream about through hard work, honesty, generosity, and avoiding the naysayers. She and her husband, Ken, befriended me when I knew no one in my new position at Johnson & Johnson. Our friendships deepened during Ken's illness and death. I cannot thank her enough for her bravery and decision to share his story.

Occasionally patients truly change how a

doctor practices medicine. This was the case with Lindsay Nohr Beck, my young patient who viewed her cancer as a hurdle and me as a necessary ally in her quest to reclaim her life. Because of her, I listen to my patients differently and no longer embrace "trickle-down medicine" as a good model. She defines patient advocacy and has proven that patients can change their doctors and stagnant medical bureaucracies. I adore her and the passion she has for living.

The Bozof family opened their home and hearts to me at an agonizing time in their lives. Their bravery and steadfastness following the death of their son, Evan, from meningococcal meningitis helped change immunization policy nationwide. Every parent in this country is indebted to them.

I have been a physician for thirty years and have been quite fortunate to weave the professions of pediatrics, surgery, and medical reporting together. During these decades I have met the most extraordinary everyday people who have shared their stories, illnesses, families, and homes. I have met world-class physicians from a multitude of countries who have taken the time to explain medical breakthroughs and advances that have truly made patients' lives better. Without patients and doctors, viewers, and friends, this project could not have come to fruition. My heartfelt thanks to all.

CONTENTS

INTRODUCTION

I don't know about you, but I like it here. Sure, life can get complicated, hard to get through, and it's not always fun, but I don't want to be shown the door anytime soon. If there are ways I can enhance my health and longevity with healthy habits, if there are appropriate screening measures for my age group, if there are new lifesaving treatments I can access, then I want to know about them so that I can stay around and be kicking up my heels when I'm ninety.

But there is a challenge you and I face: to stay healthy and live longer we need to understand and evaluate "medical myths" and learn to act on the truths behind them. Dictionaries define *myths* as widely held but mistaken beliefs, misconceptions, or misrepresentations of the truth, or exaggerated conceptions of people and institutions. Myths are like smokescreens. They prevent us from focusing clearly on the real issues and options, and most of the time we are unaware of the degree to which they shape our thoughts and guide our actions. In *Medical Myths That Can Kill You — And the 101 Truths That Will Save, Extend, and Improve Your Life,* I'll help you figure out what is true, what isn't, and how to punch holes in myths you've come to believe.

Perhaps you have been told to not go outside without wearing a coat because you'll catch pneumonia, or that you can catch a sexually transmitted disease from a toilet seat, or you'll swallow your tongue if you have a seizure. Or, more seriously, perhaps you have an elderly relative who suffered a debilitating stroke, and at thirty-something you tell yourself, "Thank God, I'm young. That can't happen to me."

Myths like these have been passed down through the ages, told and retold to us by our parents and other family members. Some were born from ancient, observed associations between the forces of nature and bodily conditions (colds and flu are more common in cold weather, for example); others are cherry-picked from the Internet. My favorite Internet myth is the one claiming that swilling cold water after a meal promotes cancer. According to this myth, the cold beverage congeals any fat you've just eaten, slowing down your digestion. This "sludge" supposedly mixes with stomach acid, is dismantled, then absorbed by the intestines where, inexplicably, it triggers cancer.

Some myths are of our own making. Human nature demands an explanation, so when the timing seems right we assume the cause of an ailment is whatever preceded it. This probably explains why so many people with achy joints chalk up their pain to humidity, storms, and any change in atmospheric pressure. This medical myth arises from our tendency to look for patterns in random events. If it rains and our joints hurt, we attribute the pain to the weather, forgetting about all the times it rained and nothing ached.

Myths are often a fusion of common sense and half-truths, which makes the truth harder to suss out. Sure, it's a good idea to bundle up before going out in the cold, but this has nothing to do with catching a cold or pneumonia, since a cold is caused by a virus and most pneumonia by bacteria. (And to answer the earlier myths: Anatomically, it's impossible to swallow your tongue if you have a seizure, since it is fastened to the floor of your mouth. And you can't catch a sexually transmitted disease from a toilet seat.

The chances of this happening are zilch, since these diseases are spread mostly through sexual intercourse.)

Some myths are more true than false. For instance, we've all heard that women's menstrual cycles echo the cycles of the moon. Is this true or false? This one is mostly true, with the walls of the uterus waxing and waning in the same rhythm as that of the celestial body in the sky. We also know that women today, as well as those in ancient times, who live and work in close proximity cycle together. It happens in the home with mothers and daughters and in the workplace with co-workers.

The fact of our bodily rhythms, whether hourly, monthly, or daily, has ushered in the exciting field of "chronotherapy" — the practice of giving a drug to a patient, according to the time of day, month, and year, as well as to phases of the sleep or menstrual cycles, in order to boost its power. Chronotherapy considers a person's biological rhythms in determining the timing — and often the dosage — of a drug to maximize its benefits and minimize its side effects. It is being studied in many different diseases, including asthma, arthritis, heart disease, and cancer.

Some myths are downright silly, others are

quite harmful, with a decidedly dark side, but all are worth our examination. Why? Knowing the difference between the reality and the myth can make your life better and even save it; there's just no doubt about it. When was the last time you heard, and maybe believed, that a heart attack can be survived by "coughing repeatedly and very vigorously" until the paramedics arrive? That you can't exercise if you have diabetes? That just because something is natural means it's safe and free of side effects? That medicines for cholesterol will damage your liver, so you shouldn't take them? Or that only women need to be concerned about bone health?

Fortunately, some medical myths just fade away when they are refuted with incontrovertible proof that shows us how to effectively treat or in some cases cure a disease. For example, when I was a resident we believed that if a kid got a fever it was a sign of a healthy immune system. The body was "cooking" the virus or the bacteria out of the body. We lived by the myth that it was better to let the fever just "run its course."

That was then. Today, an overwhelming body of medical evidence suggests that inflammatory processes like fevers, swelling, sunburn, lingering infections, or obvious inflammation-related conditions, such as asthma or rheumatoid arthritis, may be laying the groundwork for brutal illnesses never previously associated with inflammation — such as heart disease, Alzheimer's, diabetes, even cancer. Although inflammation is the body's attempt to heal, every time you have an inflammatory process going on, there is some wear and tear also occurring, not unlike having a little rusting happening inside your body. Over the long haul, that rust is harmful. So it just makes sense to manage the inflammation — which you can do not only with medicine but also through specific lifestyle changes involving exercise and diet that have been shown to keep your body as inflammation-free as possible.

Medical myths — and there are thousands of them — are alive and well in our culture. In writing this book, I distilled medical mythology down to seven of the most common — and dangerous — myths regarding our health, medical care, and longevity.

On the flip side of this, I'll give you 101 medical truths — tips, advice, and the latest scoop on how to enhance your health and save your life. These are sprinkled throughout the text, and many of these came as questions my patients have brought to me for explanation during my more than thirty

20

years as a doctor. I will also give you "news you can use" — vital medical information straight from the headlines that will help you chart and steer your own course to a healthier life.

I will explain all these myths, truths, and news to you as I have to my patients and to the viewers I reach through my job as a television medical correspondent. In this book I promise that you'll read vital medical information in a plain, practical, and straightforward manner. When you need things simplified, or when you're inundated with too much information, this book can serve as your translation guide to the now-complicated world of medicine, and I'll be your interpreter. You'll also get an insider's view of how doctors think and talk, so you can understand our language and what it means to you. Knowing this information is one vital way to keep yourself on a healthy course — for a lifetime.

Two of our greatest enemies in the battle against life-threatening diseases are ignorance and the personal beliefs we bring into the doctor's office. Are there myths you believe and hold dear? Are there old wives' tales you trust? Being willing to shift your thinking and embrace new ideas may not completely eradicate your disease risk, but

21

they may be the first steps toward making changes in your life that will. This book will give you the medical information you need to help you make informed decisions about how to:

- Get connected to the process of your own health care (yes, there is a process) — what tests, screenings, and vaccinations you need to stay healthy — and make health decisions that will benefit you most.
- Demand respect and appropriate treatment from a health-care system that isn't always fair.
- Prevent and treat the three leading causes of death in men and women — heart disease, cancer, and stroke — through awareness, self-care, prevention, and treatment.
- Learn to reverse controllable risk factors and potentially add seven years of healthy living to your life.
- Discover how a healthy mind influences a healthy body, so that you can stay well, remain active, and get the most out of your life.

Understanding medical myths clears the way to the truth and helps you see what you need to do for yourself to live a healthier, happier, and more fulfilled life. Along the way, you'll discover there are plenty of health issues over which you have a lot more control than you think. The more you know, the more prepared you are, and the better your underlying health — the better your chances of surviving *any* medical challenge thrown your way.

This book isn't a big essay or opinion piece on medical myths — on every page, there's advice and a plan of action to help you get the most out of the life you are living. It will help you treat your body as a loving friend, with enough information to help you change the habits that have plagued you up till now and correct any misinformation that inadvertently may have kept you from living up to your full health potential. However you choose to use the information in this book, my intention is that you use it as an encouraging and reassuring reminder of what's important to our health — and what's not. It is my hope that what I have to say brings renewed health and energy to your life, extends it, and possibly even saves it.

MYTH #1 ...

ANNUAL CHECKUPS ARE OBSOLETE

When I talk to people around the country, I'm always surprised to find that so many men and women believe that annual physical examinations are unnecessary. Very few see their physicians on a regular basis. I realize there are some things we would just as soon not find out, like your boyfriend's or girlfriend's entire sexual history before you met them, but having ourselves checked on a regular basis is a vital step we must take. If all of us did this, diseases could be prevented or detected at an early stage when treatment is most effective — and lives would be saved. I know this from medical experience, but I also know it from personal experience.

In 1986, while a surgeon at the University of Arkansas, I was awakened very late at night by a telephone call from my father. The minute I heard his voice, I knew something was wrong. No one in my family makes calls after 9 P.M., so this was already unsettling.

25

Age sixty-three at the time, my father — a doctor who inspired me to become one — had just had his annual physical, which he still faithfully undergoes every year. He believed that he was at risk for colon cancer, since his father had died from it in his sixties. So every year at his annual exam, Dad insisted that he get a sigmoidoscopy, the standard test back then that allowed a doctor to look at the lower part of the colon. But this time, he told his doctor he wanted a colonoscopy instead, a more thorough test that was just coming into its own. My father was convinced that this was the new standard of care and the best tool for investigation.

Today, the colonoscopy is familiar to us. With this procedure, a doctor can view the entire length of the bowel using a special telescope-like instrument called a colonoscope. For the clearest view possible, the patient flushes out the bowel the evening before using a "colon prep" of special laxatives. (I admit that the prep is no picnic, but there is no part of this test that hurts.) As it snakes its way through the bowel, the colonoscope can snare small polyps (premalignant growths) and remove them or obtain a part of a tumor for biopsy.

Although being a doctor brings me in close

proximity to life-threatening diseases, my mind went numb when Dad told me that the colonoscopy had revealed a mass, just beyond the area where the sigmoidoscopy would have stopped. There was a tumor in the wall of the colon that had eaten through and spread to two neighboring lymph nodes. A biopsy had confirmed that the mass was malignant. My dad had cancer. Because it had pierced the colon wall, I knew the situation was grim. I was stunned at how unprepared I was to deal with my father's getting a diagnosis like this. The fact that my brother and I are both surgeons didn't make this reality any easier.

But fortunately there was a happy ending. The tumor had not spread any farther than the two lymph nodes. Because radiation and chemotherapy weren't very effective for colon cancer back then, my father decided that surgery was the best treatment, and so he underwent a resection of the colon. He was right — and lucky. He has had a couple of scares since then, but twenty-one years later he has beaten cancer. Ever since it happened, he has had regular colonoscopies, every year for a while, then every two years, and now every three years. Colonoscopies aren't necessary that often for everyone, but his testing schedule reveals how individualistic exams must be. If you have had cancer, or have a strong family history of it, you and your doctor may decide that an annual look is worth it.

What happened to my friend Ken tells a different story. I first met Ken a decade ago through his wife, Andrea, with whom I had worked at Johnson & Johnson. Ken and Andrea were high school sweethearts. Retired from work, Ken was 5 feet 10 inches tall, low key in his demeanor, and a handsome man with kind eyes behind rimless glasses. His business was sales and marketing; his hobbies were rose gardening, bicycle riding, train collecting, woodworking, and Civil War history. When we shook hands, his grip was gentle but his skin rough, a casualty of his hobbies.

Ken was good about seeing his doctor but not so good about following up on required tests. He was of the mind-set that if you don't do it, then the worst couldn't and wouldn't happen. By age fifty-eight he had not had a colonoscopy. Either it went undiscussed between Ken and his doctor or Ken refused to have one — Andrea doesn't know. But when his doctor discovered through a routine blood test that Ken was anemic, the issue was forced.

Ken was suffering from iron-deficiency

TRUTH

Introduced in 1988, dual-energy X-ray absorptiometry (DEXA) technology has become a widely used tool for measuring bone density, the amount of mineral in any given area of bone. Results from bone density tests are used to diagnose osteopenia, low bone mineral density (which is in reality a sign of normal aging), and osteoporosis, in which bone density is so low that bones are prone to fracture.

You're diagnosed with osteopenia if your T-score deviates 1.0 to 2.4 points below the norm, which is the bone status of a healthy thirty-year-old. Anywhere below 2.5 standard deviations is considered osteoporosis. When you are measured against the average bone mineral density for your age group, sex, weight, and ethnic or racial origin, it is called a Z-score. However, T-scores are the gold standard for diagnosis. This means that eventually everyone's T-scores will stray from the norm, and a person with natural, age-

29

Truth, *continued*

related bone loss might appear to be suffering from osteoporosis.

There are a number of limitations to DEXA scans. One is that although these machines measure bone mineral, DEXAs do not capture information on something known as the collagen-to-mineral ratio. Too much mineral makes bones brittle; too much collagen makes them weak. Having this information would give us a better clue as to the quality of a person's bones.

DEXA scanners are not all the same, either. Bone mineral density measurements may vary markedly among machines made by different manufacturers. This means you might have normal bone density according to one machine and osteopenia according to another.

Another problem with bone density tests is that no two people are alike, even though the test holds them to the same norm. A larger-boned person may have more bone mass, thus more minerals, and may score a higher bone density than a smaller-boned person. Other variables like your genetics and your peak bone mass when you were in your twenties affect your ideal bone density. The spectrum of normal bone density is wider than this test would have you believe — which can make the test results misleading.

What concerns many of us doctors is that people are too quick to change their behavior when they think their bones are weak and porous. When a scan indicates low bone density, they feel alarmed and fragile. Often people stop lifting weights and exercising for fear of a fracture — when that's just what they need to be doing to strengthen their bones! They also may be prescribed a course of osteoporosis drugs when they don't really need them.

I approach bone density testing with a healthy dose of skepticism. For these tests to be precise, you would need to know your own baseline bone density at age twenty-five to thirty and compare it thirty years later with a reading from the same machine.

Until bone density tests become more reliable, follow your doctor's advice. Most medical experts agree that women over age sixty-five are at the highest risk for bone loss and should be tested. Your doc-

Truth, *continued*

tor may advise testing if you are younger than sixty-five and have risk factors for osteoporosis, including family history, cigarette smoking, menopause, and long-term use of medications such as steroids, thyroid medication, diuretics, and antacids containing aluminum, among others.

anemia — a form of anemia that occurs when the blood does not have enough red blood cells or does not have enough hemoglobin, a pigment in red blood cells that carries oxygen. One cause of this anemia can be slow, persistent bleeding inside the body, sometimes from tumors in the colon or elsewhere. Anemia, never a condition to be taken lightly, prompted Ken's physician to order a colonoscopy.

Ken and Andrea were on vacation when they received the news: the test uncovered colon cancer.

In the worst possible turn of events, Ken was told that his cancer was advanced. It had metastasized and set up shop in other organs. The cloud of cancer hung over Ken and Andrea for a few more years, despite multiple surgeries, chemotherapy, and radiation to try to hold it at bay. I remember being at their home, observing how painful it was for him to see the roses in his garden and not have the energy to tend to them. "Maybe I'll get to see them bloom this spring. Maybe I won't," he said quietly. Toward the end, Ken wanted only to be at home with his wife and children in a place he loved, a charming town in the Pacific Northwest tucked between snowcapped mountains and a shimmering, serene lake. Ken died at age sixty-one, three years after his diagnosis, on a February afternoon, with Andrea and his children at his bedside.

When I heard the news, I kept replaying the sequence of events in my mind. What if Ken had undergone a screening colonoscopy at age fifty? What difference would that eight years have made? If there had been a tumor, would it have been a tiny polyp — something that could have been snipped off? Would he still be here today, tending to his roses and to his family?

I have told these contrasting stories many times to many people — to my friends and loved ones, to my patients, to my students, and to my colleagues. The details that distinguished one man's experience from another's unveil an important truth: screenings and tests can mean the difference between

TRUTH

First, let me explain what a full-body scan is. This fifteen-minute, noninvasive procedure uses high-speed computed tomography (CT) to provide detailed three-dimensional images of all the major organs, including the heart, lungs, spine, and liver. It is generally available only to those willing to pay the cost: $650 to $1,500 out of their own pockets. Insurers don't routinely cover this type of screening unless it's ordered to investigate specific symptoms.

Even if you have enough money to undergo one of these scans, should you?

Probably not. In all likelihood, the scan will find an abnormality, which may actually be a "normality" for you or something quite benign — but over which you are likely to experience significant trepidation and anxiety. You will rush your report to your doctor, who will then be charged with interpreting whether the abnormality is serious or inconsequential. You'll be subjected to further tests — and further anxiety.

Even if the scan finds you in the clear, this may give you a false sense of security and possibly prevent you from seeking appropriate care from your doctor or beginning beneficial lifestyle changes. Someone who smokes, for example, and gets a clear lung scan may decide that it's okay to keep on smoking. Also, full-body scans are not a substitute for an annual checkup or appropriate screening tests.

Nor does a full-body scan find everything. For instance, it cannot pick up many debilitating and deadly conditions — like elevated blood pressure, high blood sugar, hormonal disturbances, leukemias, or abnormal cholesterol levels. Please note, too, that full-body scans are performed without intravenous dye or "contrast" injections, thereby providing limited information about the abdomen and pelvis, so small lesions in the liver, pancreas, and kidneys can be missed.

Some professional organizations, including the American College of Radiology, oppose full-body scanning as a screening tool for people with no disease

Truth, *continued*

symptoms or family history of a diagnosable problem. Further, the U.S. Food and
Drug Administration has raised concerns
about radiation levels.

There's no doubt that CT scans offer
great potential as screening tools. But
they do expose you to radiation that far
exceeds that of a routine chest X-ray. They
provide useful snapshots of the coronary
arteries, and for heavy smokers, lung
scans are excellent at pinpointing tumors.
Someday they may even replace more invasive tests. But in my opinion we're just
not there yet. Other medical tests are
much more conclusive.

life and death. The annual checkup is by no
means obsolete. It is an important step we
must all take, if for no other reason than to
make decisions with our doctors about what
screenings and tests are right for us. The appropriate scenario for screening depends on
our age, risk factors, or symptoms. Whether
we take the next step and follow through on
those recommendations is our choice, but it
is a choice that may set our compass toward
living or dying.

ANATOMY OF A MYTH

Why has the annual physical become such a debatable issue? For most of the twentieth century, the annual "head-to-toe" checkup for adults was the standard of care. Its purpose: to find disease early and reduce a person's risk of death. Then, as now, it involved blood tests, urinalysis, and screenings like chest X-rays and sometimes electrocardiograms. With the evolution of medical technology came bigger price tags, cost/benefit ratios, and public discussion of who will pay for what. Somewhere in the middle of all this, the patient — you and me — got lost. So by the late seventies, we found ourselves living in a new world of medicine. The costs of health care had skyrocketed, and in response there was a nationwide shift to managed care, in which insurers and HMOs (health maintenance organizations) began to figure out what services they could afford to offer and which ones had to go. The growing pressure on doctors to economize dictated that fewer tests be given and the cheapest treatments be offered. The yearly checkup fell under scrutiny, and several authoritative medical groups felt that healthy people didn't need physicals every year. One of these groups, the U.S. Preventive Services Task Force, an expert panel set up by Congress, feels that there isn't enough evidence that annual checkups prevent disease. Instead, these experts advise that doctors do less extensive exams in the course of a patient's care and tailor them to a person's age, sex, family background, clinical history, habits like smoking and drinking, and other risk factors. They also maintain that procedures and tests be limited to those of proven preventive value, including mammography, Pap smears, cholesterol screening, and colon cancer screening.

What do we, the doctors on the front line who are treating the healthy and those in the grip of illness, say to all this? Our response has been summed up handily in a survey published in the *Archives of Internal Medicine* in 2005. It revealed that 65 percent of all primary care doctors in the United States believe that such checkups *are* necessary. So you see, wherever ambiguity, controversy, or disagreement stews, a myth brews.

I side with the expert panel that it is vitally important to have regular screening procedures tailored for you. The important word here is *tailored*. Some tests are to be done routinely, such as blood sugar and blood pressure testing. But other tests are meant specifically for you and not necessarily for your spouse, your best friend, or your neigh-

TRUTH

Are you still smoking? How much do you drink? Are you having risky sex?

When doctors ask these questions, patients often lie because they're embarrassed, don't want to disappoint their physician, and fear being judged. Or they might rationalize their lie, promising themselves to fix the problem in the interim, so that the next time they're queried, they won't be lying. As doctors, we often know the truth anyway, because we're trained to be alert to symptoms and abnormalities, or we can run tests. If someone tells me she's stopped drinking but has tremors, or I smell alcohol on her breath, or elevated liver enzymes appear on a blood test, well, I know she's tried to pull one over on me.

There are two people you don't lie to, as an old but still-applicable saying goes: your priest and your doctor. If you can't be honest with your health-care provider, you're putting your health on the line. I once had a patient who was diagnosed

Truth, *continued*

with tongue cancer. After this occurred, he told me he had stopped smoking. He was shading the truth, and I knew it. (I can always tell because nicotine gets deposited on nose hairs, and I can smell the residue.) Sadly, he got another cancer in a different part of his mouth. I do not tell this story to lecture anyone; instead, it should serve as a reminder to you of how health problems can worsen if you lie to your doctor.

From time to time, you may have a health issue or medical problem that you'd rather not talk about to anyone, not even your doctor. Some questions, even when you're asking a doctor to answer them, can just feel too personal. Or you may be afraid that your doctor will judge you or dismiss you and not give you good treatment. From my years of working in the medical field, I can tell you that doctors are not judgmental; we've seen it all and one nude body is, well, just another nude body. We live in a very puritanical society that keeps us muffled in shame and secrecy and stigmatizes certain behaviors like smoking. But it is better to not keep these issues bottled up, especially since a frank discussion with your doctor may bring to light a positive solution. Remember your doctor is there to help you get better, so don't hold back on uncomfortable topics. Forget your shame or embarrassment and be honest. Being truthful just may save your life.

bor. I would hate to see the annual checkup go the way of the dinosaur. I join ranks with the many physicians in this country who find it vitally important — for many reasons, with benefits that are sometimes hard to quantify in this number-crunching era of managed care.

Why You Should Do It

For one, the annual checkup affords a chance to establish and build a relationship with a doctor — a connection that can prove vital if you are ever ill. I firmly believe this relationship is one of the most important you can have in your life. In a lot of ways, this relationship is very much like a good marriage, with the intimacy of trust, respect, chemistry, and communication. Meeting annually gives you the feeling that your doctor will be more than a temporary presence in your life, not a casual drop-in. We each deserve a relationship like this. How long we live, as well as how well we live, depends on it.

The doctor–patient relationship is a sensitive one, requiring respect and openness on both sides. I believe that most physicians try to do their jobs well and that most people understand that their M.D.s are human. When I was a young doctor, I was given an inside look into the world of a patient: I was misdiagnosed with a rare cancer. My physicians weren't at fault. An unusual infection from a tick bite masqueraded as a terminal illness. But none of us had figured out the mystery before I was on the receiving end of painful needles, cold hands, skimpy hospital gowns, a surgeon's scalpel, and anxiety-filled hours of waiting for lab reports. How I was treated, and the inevitable lapses that occurred, changed forever the way I take care of my patients.

To build a good relationship with our doctors, we must insist on clear, nonarrogant, and sensitive communication. Should you find that your doctor seems disinterested in you and doesn't seem to care about the details of your life, talks in language you can't decode, or is cold and insensitive, find another doctor. You deserve someone who is passionate about your care and whose an-

TRUTH

The secret to a long life is to stay in school.

We've all heard the theories on what it takes to live a long life: a healthy lifestyle, good genes, lack of stress, having lots of family and friends around, churchgoing, even wealth — and these things do make a difference. But what researchers have discovered, including those at the National Institute of Aging, is that the one consistent longevity variable among the population of every nation is education. The more educated people are, the longer — and healthier — are their lives, across the board. Education trumps race, and it trumps income in study after study when it comes to health and longevity. My parents are a good example. Now into their eighties and retired, they moved last year to my town, Princeton, N.J., where they are not only closer to three of their ten grandchildren but are also a part of a community that will continue to nurture their insatiable intellectual curiosity. The lesson: stay in school, and if you're older, never stop learning.

swers and explanations make sense to you. It is your body and your life, after all.

Second, your annual physical gives your doctor a sense of where your health stands from year to year. This yearly conversation can also be used as a form of self-monitoring regarding your habits and lifestyle and is one of the most important talks you can have. You may be queried about eating habits, exercise, smoking, alcohol or drug use, past health problems or symptoms, and concerns you may have. A headache, nagging cough, or diarrhea may signify nothing more than stress, a seasonal allergy, or food that didn't agree with you, but then again it could indicate something more serious. Talking to your doctor about symptoms at your annual checkup and during other appointments is better than a visit to the emergency room for a complaint that you might have been able to avoid by dealing with the problem earlier. While an annual physical does not turn over every stone — many conditions can escape detection — at least your doctor can investigate and identify a problem before it reaches crisis proportions and treat it early.

One last thought about the necessity of an annual checkup: it is an important time for revisiting family history. If you have a strong family history of certain conditions, say, heart disease, diabetes, or cancer, you are at risk for those diseases and should take precautions before you develop symptoms. Should you be possibly programmed to some disease by hereditary factors, your physician can guide you toward preventive measures, monitor you for complications, advise you on which screening tests you need — and when — and quite possibly keep the illness in question from ever darkening your life.

The admonishment to get an annual physical, followed by recommended screening procedures for your age, sex, and risk factors, is one bandwagon I know is worth jumping on. Despite the many reasons in its corner, I know it can be scary to undergo tests, but remember, having ourselves checked on a regular basis is the first line of defense in terms of early detection and monitoring of disease. If every person in the United States did this, more than one half of the heart disease and nearly 90 percent of many cancers in this country could be prevented or cured.

Why are we so reticent about seeing our doctors? Most of us avoid going to the physician because we can't seem to carve out the time. And when we get the time, we worry about what the doctor might find. We all hate bad news. And for some of us, the fear of worst-case scenarios is enough to make us stay away.

DON'T BE LIKE ME

On a leisurely Saturday a short while ago, I developed the worst headache, my heart started racing, and I felt like I could not catch my breath. Bone weary and pooped, I had that can't-get-out-of-bed exhaustion. No pain pills would make the headache go away. I decided to just lie down for a nap (something I rarely do) and ended up staying in bed for almost three days. My heart would race, but when I checked my pulse, my heart rate was only 66. I found myself lying there, waging an internal argument with myself.

"You're having a heart attack."

"Don't be stupid. You don't have any chest pain, and there isn't a family history."

"You know you don't have to have classic chest pain to be in trouble. Call someone."

"Wow. Look at those cobwebs on the ceiling fan."

It wasn't until the following week, when I was short of breath running up some steps, that I fully admitted something was wrong. It was my father who insisted that I see a doctor. I can still hear his words: "You know,

TRUTH

I used to try to drink eight glasses of water a day — I even recommended it to my patients — but ultimately ended up losing count or spent all my time in the bathroom. So I was happy to discover in 2002 when reading the *American Journal of Physiology* that there's no scientific study to support this recommendation. Researchers performed an exhaustive literature search and discovered that large quantities of water are not needed and that thirst regulates our water intake quite well. Our hydration needs can be met through a variety of sources in addition to drinking water. For example, we get water from juice, milk, coffee, tea, fruits, vegetables, and other foods and beverages as well. (Coffee, incidentally, is not really a diuretic. The stimulant effect of coffee produces a very slight amount of water loss. The overall volume of water you take in from your cup of coffee more than makes up for the small amount lost in your urine.)

Truth, *continued*

There's no question that water is important. It transports nutrients, hormones, and oxygen to your cells and takes away waste products via the bloodstream and lymphatic system. Water also lubricates your joints and makes you feel better. That said, how much water should you drink? Let your thirst guide you. Then look at your urine from time to time. If it's dark yellow or brown, you're dehydrated. You want to take in enough fluid each day to keep your urine looking clear like . . . water.

you're over fifty. Things can happen."

But . . . could there really be a problem with my heart? Should I see a doctor? Right now? Next week? What would happen if I waited?

There were two people warring inside me: One thought nothing of the symptoms; of course I was tired — after all, I had too much crammed on my plate, and on some days the long hours I kept blurred the transition from day to night. The other — the doctor in me — said, "I think you are having some kind of vascular crisis." Ordinarily, I would scoff at any medical person who was so wishy-washy. But I just couldn't find it in me to think that something could be wrong with my heart. No, no, no . . . I am not having a heart attack because there is no history of heart disease in my family. I'm just tired. I'll be fine. This will go away.

But the doctor-me kept up a relentless monologue, so I turned to Mary Ann, a friend and colleague who is an acclaimed internal medicine specialist and cardiologist, for help. I went in to her office sheepishly and almost apologetically (sound familiar?) and described my symptoms. Intuitively, I knew that if I hesitated any further in seeking help, I ran the risk of causing irreparable damage to my heart, if this was a heart problem at all. I kept remembering that heart disease is more often fatal in women than in men because it is frequently diagnosed at an advanced stage.

After reminding me that I knew all the warning signs of heart disease in women and scolding me for not coming in sooner, Mary Ann scheduled me for a stress test and an ultrasound of the heart. Those test results turned out normal. She believed that I likely had had a virus, which could have caused the headache and exhaustion, but to play it safe she recommended a CT angiogram, an exquisitely sensitive test for coronary heart disease that allows physicians to noninvasively capture images of the heart in just five heartbeats.

But here my plan diverted from hers. I was feeling better. I was buoyed by my normal results. And so I canceled the test. I gave some lame excuse about having to be home for my son, Charlie, and a snowstorm predicted to come our way. On some toddler level, I thought I would get away with it. Why? Deep down, I just wanted all of this to go away. I was scared.

Well, I had picked the wrong doctor for that nonsense. Mary Ann sat me down and bluntly challenged me about canceling the test. "So what you're telling me is that you don't love yourself enough to get this checked out? Don't you see how destructive, not to mention stupid, this decision is?"

I should confess right now that I have a problem with authority figures, and at this time there was only one authority figure in the room, and it wasn't me. I back-pedaled so fast that before I knew it, I was in the CT machine having my heart scanned.

It turned out that a routine virus probably did cause the symptoms. But I was in for a big surprise. My heart was not pumping blood through nonstick arteries. To the contrary. There were a couple of spots that looked like Velcro with some unfriendly plaque clinging on. I was fascinated by the image but wanted to throw up at the same time.

Pictures don't lie, however, and even a relatively untrained eye could see the problem: three tiny lesions in my coronary arteries. I also had a high "calcium score," a way of measuring how hard the plaque is. A high score meant I had flunked the exam, and I took it personally.

I confess, I was upset. Heart disease? I've never smoked. I'm not overweight (except for the ten extra pounds that I packed on ten years ago), and my body mass index (BMI) is normal. I'm not genetically inclined toward heart disease. This was unthinkable and nearly impossible to absorb. Heart disease doesn't just spring up overnight out of nowhere, however. Through a thousand flashbacks, I remembered how I ate in college and medical school, and the big picture suddenly made sense. All those years of subsisting on burgers and french fries, and now I'm paying for the nutritional sins of my youth. I remember feeling both angry and astonished that my own heart was quite possibly a ticking time bomb. In my brain I'm still a seventeen-year-old, but my arteries

TRUTH

The marketers of copper bracelets for treating arthritis claim that the copper is absorbed through the skin and thus helps repair joint cartilage deterioration. This has never been proven, and most of us get enough copper through our diets. One thing to beware of if you have arthritis is the notion that there is a miracle cure. There are no miracle cures for arthritis. All so-called miracle remedies rely on the nature of this disease, which almost always includes periods of remission, in which the pain vanishes. Put another way, with arthritis, the pain comes and goes. Take the copper bracelet, for example. You wear it. You have no flare-ups. You may attribute this to the bracelet, as the purveyor of this miracle cure would want you to do, but in fact this period of pain-free living is due to remission. It's better to spend your money on a lightweight, removable splint that you can use to immobilize the joint when you have a flare-up, and spend your time engaging in physical activities you enjoy when you don't.

---

told a different story. Whatever idea I had of my own immortality was rudely, painfully adjusted. I had no choice but to take greater responsibility for myself and start treating my body like a loving friend, and do so more resolutely.

Fortunately, my heart condition is easily, eminently fixable. I am now taking a cholesterol-lowering drug, joining the ranks of millions of Americans who are on statins. I said good-bye to fatty meats, resolved to get more exercise, and embraced vegetables as a formal religion. Doing this, I expect my heart condition to reverse itself.

With a DVD of my heart exam in hand (yes, you now can get DVDs of the inner workings of your body), I trotted home. It was family movie night at our house, and I insisted that everyone indulge me by watching my DVD. My family already knew I had a big heart metaphorically speaking. Now I wanted them to see the literal one, albeit a little banged up.

When I talk to my patients, I often recount

NEWS YOU CAN USE

The Ornish diet may be the best plan for heart health, say researchers at the University of Massachusetts who compared eight popular diets. Dr. Dean Ornish suggests that if you stick with a nonfat vegetarian diet, you'll lower your risk of not only heart disease but also stroke and cancer. The only problem: it's strict and can be hard to stick to long term.

this experience. It levels the playing field and lets them know that I've been a patient, too — a reluctant one at that, caught up in the same gale of fear and anxiety, likely to avoid making an appointment or keeping it.

Sure, a symptom may be nothing, but then again it may be serious. Avoidance doesn't help and may even worsen a problem. Some of us snub physicians because we've been conscientious, had clear checkups for a couple of years, feel healthy, and see this year's checkup as a waste of time. When you find yourself thinking this way, think about your car. Consider how you remember to rotate the tires and check the oil. Then think about yourself. Think of your annual physical as your forty-thousand-mile tune-up. Time consuming as it may be, having a yearly check under the hood gives your doctor the most information regarding your health and the greatest chance of diagnosing any condition as early as possible.

To stay healthy — and possibly save your life — you have to take responsibility for your body's maintenance. This includes the obvious and the boring: Watch what you eat. Don't smoke. Stop abusing alcohol or drugs. Listen to your body when it's tired, and get enough rest. Minimize stress. Exercise. In short, practice prevention before prescriptive medical measures are necessary. The other part to prevention is surveillance, which includes your annual checkup and screening for the health issues you suspect will be part of your life's road map. Take measures for your age group and risk factors. Getting in the habit of scheduling — and keeping — your medical appointments, including your annual checkup, requires some conscious effort, so here is my advice on how to do it.

RESPECT YOUR BODY

Reframe your view of the annual checkup, not as something to be feared or dismissed, but as a gift you give to yourself. Consider it a way to respect yourself and your body and take what responsibility you can for it. Think of the times you have wasted money on something frivolous, and then consider this the opposite — a deposit in the bank of better health.

Pick a special date for your annual checkup — it can be your birthday, anniversary, or any date you choose, and consider it carved in stone. This is an easy way for you to remember when to have the necessary tests done, and there's no excuse for missing them. Then, on the day you have the exam, immediately schedule next year's appointment and put it on your calendar. That way, no muss, no fuss.

Having annual checkups is not only something you do for yourself. It is also something you do for your family. I recall some-

NEWS YOU CAN USE

Lift weights and call me in the morning! Regular strength training not only firms muscles, but it also boosts your immune system and creates a faster metabolism. Stronger muscles also make your bones stronger.

TRUTH

Do you know what cyberchondriacs are?

They're people who are convinced they've caught every disease on the Web. They feel a symptom, look it up on the Internet, and diagnose themselves. Let's say your ankles are swelling. You use Google to search for "ankle swelling." Your search produces roughly 136,000 matches. An experienced cyberchondriac can make a diagnosis on the basis of just a few matching symptoms, but here you've got more matches than you could dream up illnesses to correspond. You ignore benign causes like "poorly fitting clothes" or "ankle injury" and zero in on scary stuff like heart failure instead. The symptom list for heart failure numbers at least twenty-two. Among them: fatigue, tiredness, abnormal weight gain, and of course, your swollen ankles. You decide you have all these symptoms, so you conclude you have heart failure. You then start feeling anxious and short of breath, yet

Truth, *continued*

another symptom of heart failure.

I reported on a Harris Interactive Poll recently and learned that more than 160 million of us now search for health information on the Web. Of these, 84 percent of us are cyberchondriacs, people who search for medical information on the Web at least six times a month and try to diagnose a disease prior to consulting a doctor.

I think mainstream medical websites can be a fabulous educational resource for medical information — and an educated patient is a good patient — but they also have the potential to be a big problem. Medical websites give you the ability to self-diagnose without the proper care and treatment of a medical doctor, at the risk of great harm and mental anguish. And as you've probably already heard, only fools have themselves for a doctor!

If you are trolling the Web, I would rather see you reference websites of established medical centers, medical schools, medical journals, or nonprofit research centers if you have or suspect a serious illness. But the best advice: talk to your doctor, not the Web. It can really handicap your doctor if you walk in with sheaves of medical information you've downloaded from the Internet. This limits the time your doctor has to assess your condition. Allow your doctor the time to treat you; this is what we are trained to do. Again, if you truly think you're having a serious medical problem, rather than clicking on symptoms, call your doctor. You'll get a better assessment, even over the phone. Or head straight to the emergency room or your doctor's office for medical attention.

thing my mother once so wisely told me: "Taking care of yourself is the best gift you can give your children." How true! When we care for ourselves, we are anything but self-indulgent or selfish. We are strengthening our bodies and renewing our spirit and, in the process, giving our family the very best of ourselves. My parents have always taken good care of themselves, and despite a few health scares, at the time of this writing they are in their eighties and on a hiking vacation in Scotland. They look and act much younger than their years, and they have themselves to thank for it.

BE AN INFORMED PATIENT

Become informed about the recommended tests appropriate for your age, sex, and risk factors. Medical tests fall into two broad categories: screening and diagnostic. Screening tests are the first line of defense in terms of identifying health problems at an early stage, often before they cause any symptoms. There are many kinds of tests that qualify as screening tests, from clinical breast exams, mammography, PSA tests, Pap smears, exercise tests, and imaging tests. Diagnostic tests, on the other hand, help us confirm or deny the presence of health problems.

Test results, in general, are initially interpreted by "invisible doctors" like radiologists or pathologists, whom you rarely see, and the results are passed along to your doctor, who in turn interprets them to you. If this all sounds suspiciously like the kids' game of rumor, where information is whispered from one child to the next, distorted along the way until it comes out as one hilarious garbled mess, relax — it's not that bad. Even so, I'm a big believer in having patients understand their own lab and pathology reports, because the more interpretation that goes on, the more room there is for error. There is nothing so complicated or technical in these reports that it cannot be explained to or understood by you, given lucid clarification by your doctor. It is very appropriate for you to ask your physician to fully explain your test results in terms you can comprehend. Such dialogue should be embraced by a doctor; it gives your physician a chance to know you even better.

As we age there are more reasons to see the doctor on a regular basis than there may have been when we were younger. If you have certain conditions — high blood pressure, a high LDL cholesterol level, diabetes, ulcers or other digestive disorders — you'll know what kind of schedule you should be keeping and what specialized tests you might need.

With the heart-attack-like symptoms I experienced recently, my doctor advised a CT angiogram. It is a specialized test that isn't necessary that often, unless symptoms warrant it and your doctor wants extra information. Most doctors would not consider it as standard, but without it I would not have seen inside the arteries of my heart, and I may not have been as serious about making that plaque go away. Seeing is not just believing; it's taking action. As for standard tests and screenings, the charts on pages 64–70 will give you a clearer sense of which tests may be right for you.

BECOME A PARTNER WITH YOUR PHYSICIAN

After all, this is your body — not your doctor's. Sit down and talk about the tests and decide which of them you need, in addition to your annual checkup. There is no such thing as a "routine" screening or checkup, either, since everyone is different. We all can gather information, look at our family trees and how we have lived our own lives, and forecast the reality of what may lie ahead. If it's too much to think about all at once, sit down and make a list of the diseases or conditions for which you may be at risk — and those you have now. Put pen to paper and take a few days to be thorough. Talk to your doctor about what tests should be individualized to your needs and at what age you should start getting them.

Because my father was diagnosed with colon cancer and my grandfather died of it, I have had regular colonoscopies since turning forty, as have my siblings. The first time I had one, my doctor found an abnormal polyp and removed it. It wasn't cancer, but I believe it was headed in that direction. Each year on my birthday, I schedule the necessary battery of tests — a physical, a pelvic exam, a mammogram. Doing this has given me a sense that I have controlled the aspects of my life that I can. Every three years, I have a colonoscopy. Again, that may be too often for some of you and not often enough for others, but that's my point. I get what I need — what I believe will keep this chassis and engine going. So I feel very comfortable with the screening procedures I have outlined for myself, and I believe you have to be just as comfortable with whatever you and your doctor establish for you.

PREPARE FOR YOUR ANNUAL CHECKUP AND OTHER VISITS TO THE DOCTOR

Jot down questions and concerns: *I have periodic headaches. Is this a sign of tension, a hormone imbalance, an injury, or some other*

MEDICAL TESTS AND SCREENINGS FOR WOMEN				
Screening Tests	Ages 18 to 39	Ages 40 to 49	Ages 50 to 64	Ages 65 and Older
General health Full checkup, including weight and height	Annually	Annually	Annually	Annually
Thyroid TSH test	Start at age 35, then every 5 years	Every 5 years	Every 5 years	Every 5 years
Heart health Blood pressure test	At every appointment, more often if your blood pressure is elevated	At every appointment, more often if your blood pressure is elevated	At every appointment, more often if your blood pressure is elevated	At every appointment, more often if your blood pressure is elevated

Screening Tests	Ages 18 to 39	Ages 40 to 49	Ages 50 to 64	Ages 65 and Older
Cholesterol test	Start at age 20, then every 5 years or at your doctor's discretion; if your total cholesterol is above 200, you should be tested more often.	Every 5 years or at your doctor's discretion; if your total cholesterol is above 200, you should be tested more often.	Every 5 years or at your doctor's discretion; if your total cholesterol is above 200, you should be tested more often.	Every 5 years or at your doctor's discretion; if your total cholesterol is above 200, you should be tested more often.
Bone health Bone density test		Discuss with your doctor or nurse.	Discuss with your doctor or nurse.	Discuss with your doctor or nurse.
Diabetes Blood glucose test	Discuss with your doctor or nurse.	Start at age 45, then every 3 years	Every 3 years	Every 3 years

MEDICAL TESTS AND SCREENINGS FOR WOMEN				
Screening Tests	Ages 18 to 39	Ages 40 to 49	Ages 50 to 64	Ages 65 and Older
Breast health Doctor's breast exam	Annually	Annually	Annually	Annually
Self-exams	Monthly	Monthly	Monthly	Monthly
Mammogram (X-ray of breast)		Every 1 to 2 years. Discuss with your doctor or nurse.	Every 1 to 2 years. Discuss with your doctor or nurse.	Every 1 to 2 years. Discuss with your doctor or nurse.
Reproductive health Pap test and pelvic exam	Every 1 to 3 years if you have been sexually active or are older than 21	Every 1 to 3 years	Every 1 to 3 years	Discuss with your doctor or nurse.

Chlamydia test	Annually until age 25 if sexually active. Older than age 25, get this test if you have new or multiple partners. All pregnant women should have this test.	Get this test if you have new or multiple partners. All pregnant women should have this test.	Discuss with your doctor or nurse.	Discuss with your doctor or nurse.
Sexually transmitted disease (STD) tests	Both partners should get tested for STDs, including HIV, before initiating sexual intercourse.	Both partners should get tested for STDs, including HIV, before initiating sexual intercourse.	Both partners should get tested for STDs, including HIV, before initiating sexual intercourse.	Both partners should get tested for STDs, including HIV, before initiating sexual intercourse.

MEDICAL TESTS AND SCREENINGS FOR WOMEN				
Screening Tests	Ages 18 to 39	Ages 40 to 49	Ages 50 to 64	Ages 65 and Older
Colorectal health				
Fecal occult blood test			Annually	Annually
Colonoscopy			Every 10 years or as directed	Every 10 years or as directed
Rectal exam	Discuss with your doctor or nurse.	Discuss with your doctor or nurse.	Every 5 to 10 years with each screening (colonoscopy)	Every 5 to 10 years with each screening (colonoscopy)

Eye and ear health			
Eye exam	If you have any visual problems; or at least one exam from ages 20 to 29 and at least two exams from ages 30 to 39.	Every 2 to 4 years	Every 2 to 4 years	Every 1 to 2 years
Hearing test	Starting at age 18, then every 10 years	Every 10 years	Every 3 years	Every 3 years
Skin health			
Mole exam	Monthly mole self-exam; by a doctor every 3 years, starting at age 20.	Monthly mole self-exam; by a doctor annually.	Monthly mole self-exam; by a doctor annually.	Monthly mole self-exam; by a doctor annually.

MEDICAL TESTS AND SCREENINGS FOR WOMEN					
Screening Tests	Ages 18 to 39	Ages 40 to 49	Ages 50 to 64	Ages 65 and Older
Oral health Dental exam	One to two times every year	One to two times every year	One to two times every year	One to two times every year
Abdominal Aortic aneurysm test				Annually, if you are older than 65 and have a history of heart disease or smoking; have a screening test, which looks for any abnormally large or swollen blood vessels in your abdomen.

Adapted from National Women's Health Information Center, www.4woman.gov/screeningscharts/general.htm.

70

condition? I'm not sleeping well. Should I take some sort of medication? I have some moles that seem to be changing. Should I see a specialist? My bowel habits are irregular. Is there a test I should have? Also, bring in a list of all medications you're taking — including prescription medicines, over-the-counter drugs, and dietary supplements you are currently on or have stopped taking within the last month. List how often you take them and what dosages. If a medication or treatment isn't working, let your doctor know so that he or she can take corrective action. If you are presently seeing other doctors, take along a list of their names, addresses, and telephone numbers.

IT'S OKAY TO FEEL WORRIED

Finally, keep in mind that it is perfectly normal to feel anxiety regarding the outcome of your checkups, screenings, and other medical tests. Don't let anyone convince you that you're neurotic. You're not. We all wait for the results of tests with some degree of trepidation. If you can keep your nerves intact, more power to you. Just try to relax and occupy your time with other matters. The odds are in your favor that everything will be fine. Just remember what a chicken I was. I know you can be much braver!

MEDICAL TESTS AND SCREENINGS FOR MEN				
Screening Tests	Ages 18 to 39	Ages 40 to 49	Ages 50 to 64	Ages 65 and Older
General health Full checkup, including weight and height	Annually	Annually	Annually	Annually
Heart health Blood pressure test	At every appointment, more often if your blood pressure is elevated	At every appointment, more often if your blood pressure is elevated	At every appointment, more often if your blood pressure is elevated	At every appointment, more often if your blood pressure is elevated

Cholesterol test	Start at age 20, then every 5 years or at your doctor's discretion; if your total cholesterol is above 200, you should be tested more often.	Every 5 years or at your doctor's discretion; if your total cholesterol is above 200, you should be tested more often.	Every 5 years or at your doctor's discretion; if your total cholesterol is above 200, you should be tested more often.	Every 5 years or at your doctor's discretion; if your total cholesterol is above 200, you should be tested more often.
Diabetes Blood glucose test	Discuss with your doctor or nurse.	Start at age 45, then every 3 years	Every 3 years	Every 3 years
Prostate health Digital rectal exam (DRE)		Discuss with your doctor or nurse.	Annually, starting at age 50	Annually

MEDICAL TESTS AND SCREENINGS FOR MEN				
Screening Tests	Ages 18 to 39	Ages 40 to 49	Ages 50 to 64	Ages 65 and Older
Prostate-specific antigen (PSA) blood test		Discuss with your doctor or nurse.	Annually, starting at age 50	Annually
Reproductive health Testicular exam	Monthly self-exam; and part of a general checkup.	Monthly self-exam; and part of a general checkup.	Monthly self-exam; and part of a general checkup.	Monthly self-exam; and part of a general checkup.
Chlamydia test	Discuss with your doctor or nurse.	Discuss with your doctor or nurse.	Discuss with your doctor or nurse.	Discuss with your doctor or nurse.

74

Sexually trans-mitted disease (STD) tests	Both partners should get tested for STDs, includ-ing HIV, before initiating sexual intercourse.	Both partners should get tested for STDs, includ-ing HIV, before initiating sexual intercourse.	Both partners should get tested for STDs, including HIV, before initiating sexual intercourse.
Colorectal health Fecal occult blood test			Annually
Colonoscopy		Every 10 years or as directed	Every 10 years or as directed
Rectal exam	Discuss with your doctor or nurse.	Every 5 to 10 years with each screening (colonoscopy)	Every 5 to 10 years with each screening (colonoscopy)

75

MEDICAL TESTS AND SCREENINGS FOR MEN				
Screening Tests	Ages 18 to 39	Ages 40 to 49	Ages 50 to 64	Ages 65 and Older
Eye and ear health				
Eye exam	If you have any visual problems; or at least one exam from ages 20 to 29 and at least two exams from ages 30 to 39.	Every 2 to 4 years	Every 2 to 4 years	Every 1 to 2 years
Hearing test	Starting at age 18, then every 10 years	Every 10 years	Discuss with your doctor or nurse.	Discuss with your doctor or nurse.

Skin health Mole exam	Monthly mole self-exam; by a doctor every 3 years, starting at age 20.	Monthly mole self-exam; by a doctor annually.	Monthly mole self-exam; by a doctor annually.	Monthly mole self-exam; by a doctor annually.
Oral health Dental exam	One to two times every year	One to two times every year	One to two times every year	One to two times every year

MEDICAL TESTS AND SCREENINGS FOR MEN				
Screening Tests	Ages 18 to 39	Ages 40 to 49	Ages 50 to 64	Ages 65 and Older
Abdominal Aortic aneurysm test				Annually, if you are older than 65 and have a history of heart disease or smoking; have a screening test, which looks for any abnormally large or swollen blood vessels in your abdomen.

Adapted from National Women's Health Information Center, www.4woman.gov/screeningscharts/men.

TRUTH

Drug mistakes are a leading cause of death and illness in this country.

Medication errors are among the most common medical mistakes, harming at least 1.5 million people every year and killing approximately 7,000 people annually, according to the Institute of Medicine, an independent, nonprofit organization that advises the federal government on health issues. Is there something you, as a patient, can do to avoid medication errors? You bet.

If your doctor has prescribed medication for you, be sure you understand what you're taking and why. Ask questions — including what to expect. For example: What is the name of the drug, and is there a generic version available that might save money? What is the medication supposed to do? What is the dosage? What are the side effects, both physical and psychological? What should I do if side effects occur? How will the medication improve my condition? How long will it take to work? How will it interact with

Truth, *continued*

other drugs, food, or other substances? Don't be embarrassed to take notes while the doctor is talking. Or bring a friend or loved one to help you take down the information you need, if you're feeling overwhelmed. And if you are seeing more than one doctor, make sure that your primary doctor knows what all your other M.D.s are prescribing.

Be sure you understand the written material that comes with the drug and on its label. This is tricky. If you've read the warning labels on medicines and health-care products, you will know what I mean. Ambien (a sleeping pill), for instance, carries a warning that says "might make you drowsy." One tampon package advises, "Remove used tampon before inserting new one." I do not know whether I should thank the companies that produced these products for their touching concern for my health or send a letter asking them what they think my IQ is. As you do with your doctor, ask your pharmacist to explain how to properly take the drug, its side effects, and what to do if you experience any.

TRUTH

While you were growing up, your mother probably practiced medicine on you: "Don't read in the dark or you'll go blind!" Not true. You won't damage your eyes by using them. Reading in low light will not change the health or function of your eyes. You'll see better if the lighting is optimal, but dim light has no permanent effect on the structure of your eyes.

Even so, reading in dim light can lead to temporary eyestrain. So find a good lamp, and keep your reading material at least twelve inches away from your eyes. Then take a break from reading every twenty minutes or so to give your eyes a rest.

Blinking keeps your eyes wet and clears away dust. So try to blink more often when you feel your eyes getting tired. And if you want to help your eyes and beautify your home at the same time, try adding a few houseplants. Plants increase the air's humidity, which is good for your eyes.

Poor eyesight can also lead to eyestrain. So, if you have glasses, remember to wear them.

TRUTH

Sunglasses aren't just a fashion statement; they also protect your eyes from harmful ultraviolet light. Exposure to sunlight is the leading cause of cataracts in the United States, and cataracts are the leading cause of blindness among elderly Americans. In people over 65, cataract surgery is one of the most common operations. The disease is one reason to wear sunglasses year-round to filter out the sun's damaging UVA and UVB rays.

THE POWER OF PERSONAL INTUITION

New screening and diagnostic technologies for detecting and monitoring all forms of disease are unfolding at an extraordinary rate. Someday, for example, we'll have at our disposal highly precise scans capable of picking up once-unseen abnormalities. Someday, we'll have prenatal tests that will generate a genetic profile of our unborn child so that diseases can be genetically modified and treated before they ever manifest. Someday,

cancer may be as easy to detect as high cholesterol, thanks to highly sophisticated blood
tests that through "biomarkers" (micro-
scopic footprints of cancer in the bloodstream) will be able to find this dreaded disease long before it is big enough to do any
damage. There's no question that technology
is progressing in time to bring us new and
better ways to do our medical detective
work. But we cannot rely solely on technology as our savior.

A diagnosis, a treatment plan, or any sort
of doctor's orders are built not only from a
physician's knowledge of how to treat disease but also from what you openly and honestly convey during appointments. As a
physician, I know that the majority of illnesses are first detected or, better yet, felt or
intuited by you, the patient. You know yourself, and you know what normal well-being
is for you. You are much better off if you pay
attention to what you see, what you feel, and
what you sense in your own body.

In June 2007 I covered a medical report on
ovarian cancer, one of the scariest cancers
around. It kills more women than all other
gynecologic cancers combined, and until
then we believed there were no early warning
signs. This was not a story about some high-
tech, state-of-the-art screening test; this was

TRUTH

You've probably seen television commercials touting prescription drugs for something called restless leg syndrome, or RLS. And you've said to yourself, "This must be made up." Even doctors have been skeptical about it. But RLS is a medical condition. Sufferers frequently experience strong urges to move their legs, often at night, sometimes accompanied by persistent uncomfortable leg sensations. The discomfort is temporarily relieved by getting up and walking around or by moving the legs. As you might imagine, this condition does not make it easy to relax and get much sleep. Recently, researchers discovered that RLS appears to run in families and have isolated a gene that may predispose some people to developing the problem. Fortunately, RLS can be treated with two drugs, one called Requip and the other called Mirapex. Although both have side effects, most of the people who take these drugs say they're able to get a good night's sleep for the first time in years. Some people report relief with nondrug methods, too: hot baths prior to sleeping; avoiding alcohol, nicotine, and caffeine; exercising early in the day; and following a healthy diet that includes iron-rich foods such as lean meats and iron-fortified foods (since RLS is associated with iron insufficiency).

not a story about a new therapy that could cure this cancer. No, this was a story about something decidedly low tech: symptoms — the clues a woman senses in her own body.

In a first, cancer researchers announced a constellation of symptoms that might point to ovarian cancer: bloating, pelvic pain, difficulty eating, feeling full, and needing to urinate frequently. Yes, these are symptoms that could also indicate a host of other ailments, and most of the time they are nothing to worry about. But when these symptoms come and stay, lasting for two weeks or more, they could prove quite significant. They could indicate early ovarian cancer. And while there is no great screening test for cancer of the ovaries, this is one cancer where catching it early can be the difference between life and death. Early stage ovarian cancer has a 90 percent cure rate, but by the time it has spread, the cure rate drops to 20 percent. With those numbers in mind, it is imperative for a woman to listen to her body and report her symptoms to her physician. Doctors and medical experts believe that this simple act of vigilance may save many lives.

The wisdom of seeing our doctors on a regular basis, familiarizing ourselves with symptoms of serious illnesses, knowing our risk factors, and not letting anything get in the way of regular screening tests still applies and always will. I hope you're with me on this. Technology has its limits; intuition and diligence do not.

Up next is something to take up with your doctor at your next appointment. Turn the page, and you'll be reacquainted with a preventive treatment that is still saving lives every day.

MYTH #2 . . .

VACCINATIONS ARE JUST FOR KIDS

The myth of vaccinations for kids only is one I believed in until I did a report in 1999 for *20/20* about outbreaks of meningococcal meningitis on college campuses. What I heard and saw changed me as a doctor and as a mother.

Twenty-year-old Evan Bozof was a robust, handsome college student and the star pitcher for the baseball team at Georgia Southwestern University, and as a premed major, he dreamed of becoming a doctor. One day, during the spring of his junior year, Evan complained of a severe headache, accompanied by flulike symptoms. Like most college students, he had stayed up late, studying for exams and partying on the weekend. So coming down with the flu was certainly within the realm of possibility. He felt so sick that, uncharacteristically, he skipped his baseball game and had a friend take him to the emergency room. Evan

TRUTH

Affecting more than five hundred thousand adults annually, shingles (herpes zoster) is characterized by a painful rash that results from an old chicken pox infection years before. After the chicken pox clears up, the pox virus remains dormant (inactive) in nerve roots and can reemerge years later. Stress, illness, and advanced age are triggers that can activate the dormant pox virus in the nerve roots, causing shingles to erupt.

Technically, you cannot catch shingles from another person by brushing up against them. But if you have shingles, stay away from pregnant women, children, and people with compromised immune systems. The blisters do contain the chicken pox virus. If you have never had chicken pox, avoid touching someone who has shingles. Talk to your doctor about the shingles vaccine, Zostavax, if you are age sixty or older. There are also antiviral medications such as acyclovir

(Zovirax), famciclovir (Famvir), and valacy-clovir (Valtrex) that can help to get rid of shingles. These medications can also help reduce the chance of postherpetic neuralgia, a lingering pain that can develop along the nerve line of the outbreak in people over the age of fifty.

ended up in the hospital for observation instead of heading home for spring break.

The next morning, his doctors realized this wasn't a viral infection, and it sure wasn't the flu. Evan had meningococcal meningitis, a rare but potentially fatal bacterial infection that causes inflammation of the membranes surrounding the brain and spinal cord. It is a disease that strikes about three thousand Americans each year according to the U.S. Centers for Disease Control and Prevention (CDC), with nearly 12 percent of the cases resulting in death. Those who survive often face irreversible consequences such as permanent brain damage, hearing loss, or limb amputations. Approximately 100 to 125 cases occur annually on college campuses.

Within hours, a fever and a telltale rash turned to hemorrhages under Evan's skin. Hour by hour, he became sicker as the bac-

TRUTH

The original idea of "feed a cold, starve a fever" dates back to the sixteenth century when a dictionary maker wrote, "Fasting is a great remedie of feuer." His medical advice wasn't so hot, and the idea of feeding a cold and starving a fever has dogged the path of cold treatment ever since. Therefore, it's probably time to lay this old wives' tale to rest once and for all. The common cold is an illness caused by a viral infection in the nose. Symptoms include sneezing, runny nose, congestion, a sore or scratchy throat, often accompanied by headache, chills, or fever. It is a good idea to feed a cold but a bad idea to starve a fever, since your body needs nutrition at all times for healing. When your temperature goes up, so does your metabolism — which means your body requires calories more than ever to carry out basic functions like breathing and pumping blood. Not eating will only make it harder for your body to fight off the illness.

teria and their toxins proved too much for his body to fight. His blood vessels became blocked, and his fingers and toes turned blue and then black, signifying the irreversible onslaught of gangrene.

Evan's doctors sedated him and put him into a drug-induced coma to prevent uncontrollable seizures, and Evan's parents began their bedside vigil. Over the course of a gruesome two weeks, his parents made the agonizing decision to amputate a leg, then the other, and then an arm and another arm, in an attempt to save his life. His mother, Lynn, took photos so that when Evan pulled through, they'd be able to explain to him why they made the decisions that they did.

But Evan never woke up. The infection was too aggressive, and no antibiotic or medical treatment could keep pace with it. Evan died in the hospital, with his mother and father in attendance, twenty-six days after his diagnosis. His family had to deal with the most ex-

TRUTH

The biggest breeding ground for germs in your bathroom is not your hairbrush.

It's your toothbrush. We know from research that used toothbrushes are contaminated with millions of germs from our mouths, from the bathroom, and from neighboring toothbrushes. To keep germs from spreading, don't share toothbrushes or let your toothbrush make contact with any other toothbrushes stored in the same holder. A good rule of thumb is to keep them at least an inch apart. Also, get a new toothbrush after you've had any illness such as a cold or flu because germs can remain even after you've recovered. Another tip: always flush your toilet with the lid down, or move your toothbrush to inside your medicine cabinet. The reason is gross, but it's true: the spray and mist from a flushed toilet can spread as far as twenty feet. The only solution for most of us is to drop that lid before we flush. The polluted water vapor that erupts out of the flushing toilet bowl can take several hours to really settle. You get the picture by now.

> If your toothbrush is too close to the toilet, you are brushing your teeth with toilet water. Ugh.

cruciating loss a parent could ever experience.

One of the tragedies in this story is that a simple immunization, a vaccine for meningococcal meningitis, could have saved Evan's life. His mom had even asked the family doctor about it before Evan went to college and the doctor assured her that it wasn't necessary. It would have cost eighty dollars, the price of a pair of tennis shoes.

I returned home from the interview with Evan's parents, stunned by the story I had heard, the pictures I had seen, and the people I had met. In life, many circumstances are out of your hands, but this was controllable and avoidable. No one knew this better than his parents, who now have to cope every day with anguish over the needless death of their young and vibrant son.

By the time I finished working on this story, I had enough research and information about meningococcal meningitis to make a different decision. The vaccine was readily available, so I had all three of my

TRUTH

Sexually transmitted diseases, or STDs, are caught by direct contact with the bacteria or virus that is the cause of specific diseases, through vaginal or anal intercourse, or by oral–genital contact. To catch an STD from a toilet seat, you would have to have direct contact at the site on the skin with the microorganisms. It is highly improbable that this would ever occur. The bacteria and viruses that cause STDs tend to be highly sensitive to environmental conditions and can't survive outside the human body for very long, especially on hard surfaces like toilet seats.

So, if you don't want to squat anymore over the toilet seat, like your mother insisted when you were a child, you can be somewhat relieved — except for two things: You can still get wet if you sit, and that's creepy. And you could get crabs. Although not technically an STD, this form of lice can hop from a person to the toilet seat, and then to you. On second thought, I'm going to listen to my mom.

TRUTH

The worst room in your house to stockpile your medicines is the bathroom. The humidity and swings in temperature can age medications prematurely, which is why I keep the real medicines — the ones we take by mouth — in a separate area in a hall closet. If you don't have that kind of storage space, just grab one of your old shoe boxes and arrange the essentials neatly inside. But remember: if you have children or grandchildren around your home, you must keep this box out of their reach. Use your built-in medicine cabinet for things like bandages and dental floss.

children vaccinated. I've come to grips with the fact that this disease neither recognizes socioeconomic barriers nor respects how good you are at feeding your children or tucking them into bed at night. It can strike at any time and has dramatic killing power.

There was one small consolation to the Evan Bozof story. Lynn Bozof created meaning from tragedy. With other parents, she formed the National Meningitis Foundation. Its crusade is simple: get adolescents vaccinated. Today, a majority of colleges and

TRUTH

Mosquitoes are the deadliest insects on earth.

The female Anopheles mosquito is easily awarded the title "deadliest animal on earth." It is responsible for more than 300 million cases of malaria each year and causes approximately 1.2 million deaths. There are three thousand species of mosquitoes, some two hundred in North America, but they do not all transmit the same diseases. Mosquitoes also carry dengue and yellow fevers, encephalitis, elephantiasis, and canine heartworm. Mosquitoes are most active at night. You can protect yourself from bites by wearing long sleeves and insect repellent while outside. Also, be sure to empty any standing water such as birdbaths, gutters, or outdoor containers, since these can be breeding grounds for mosquitoes.

universities require the vaccine for entry. Yet still only twenty-three states mandate it for children, teens, and state-supported universities. This is not good enough.

ANATOMY OF A MYTH

I have thought about Evan Bozof many times in the years since and how his life could have been saved by a simple vaccination. I believe that vaccines are the greatest medical breakthrough of the past century. It's easy to disregard them because they no longer seem modern or jazzy. Vaccines have been with us since the days of George Washington, when the English country doctor Edward Jenner first used the pus from cowpox blisters taken from infected milkmaids to inoculate people against smallpox. That rudimentary vaccine worked and medicine was transformed. By the end of the twentieth century, we relied on vaccines to prevent many dreaded infections — among them, smallpox, which has been eradicated worldwide.

With all the modern advances we have at our disposal, it is easy to forget what life was like before the dawn of vaccinations. We can't recall polio wards and children struggling for breath from whooping cough. We don't remember the thousands of children

TRUTH

HIV, the virus that causes AIDS, is found in significant concentrations only in semen, vaginal secretions, blood, and breast milk. It is through the exchange of these body fluids that the virus can be passed from one person to another. The virus is not found in high enough concentrations in other fluids or the skin to make casual contact a concern. It is not contracted through such everyday events as shaking hands or hugging, and it is not transmitted by being exposed to someone's tears; nor is it possible to contract it through the saliva exchanged in kissing. It would take gallons and gallons of saliva to present any risk at all of infection — certainly more saliva than the most passionate of deep kissers could exchange.

who died from measles. These diseases terrified our grandparents, yet most of us will never see or experience a case. But we shouldn't forget that vaccinations are still

TRUTH

Once infected with genital herpes, you have it for life. At least a third of those infected never experience a second, noticeable case, which is why they erroneously believe they are cured and may unknowingly infect others. There are currently three antiviral therapies available for the genital herpes infection: valacyclovir (Valtrex), famciclovir (Famvir), and acyclovir (Zovirax). These prescription medications have two main roles: to treat outbreaks and, as suppressive therapy, to keep the virus at bay. There is no evidence, however, that the infection can be permanently "cured" by existing antiviral therapies.

needed — it is estimated that vaccine-preventable deaths kill as many as seventy thousand American adults every year. And new vaccines are being developed to fight a host of diseases, from new strains of germs to cancer to heart disease. So, in the interim, we need to keep up with our vaccinations and not minimize their importance.

The astounding success of vaccinations has lulled us into thinking that they are something we can opt in or out of. I was a part of the generation who lined up in the school cafeteria to have vaccine-soaked sugar cubes put in my mouth. My parents didn't get the opportunity to opt out, and there weren't permission slips. It's a very different animal today, with many pockets of

TRUTH

Stress does not cause ulcers.

Stress lays the foundation for some illnesses, but ulcers are not one of them. Ulcers are caused by a strain of bacteria called *Helicobacter*. When the medical world first heard this years ago, we thought it was a joke — until we were persuaded by an overwhelming body of scientific evidence. Nearly two-thirds of the world's population is infected with this bacteria. But fortunately, people with ulcers can be cured with antibiotics.

TRUTH

You can't catch a cold from being in cold weather.

The myth that you can catch a cold from being cold, venturing outside in the rain without an umbrella, or going out into winter weather with wet hair dies hard. Even some historians are still reporting that President William Henry Harrison caught a cold that developed into fatal pneumonia because he made his inaugural speech in the rain. He died before he had been in office a month. If you read between the lines, they're implying that had he only stayed dry, he would not have had the briefest presidency in the history of the office. The truth is that colds are caused by viruses that are transmitted from one person to another by touching something that has the virus on it, then touching your eye, nose, or mouth. Can you guess the easiest way to catch a cold? Shaking hands with someone, then putting that hand to your face.

society in the United States saying no to vaccinations, "not in my village." There is a new generation of worried parents (again, who have never seen a case of polio or measles) who question the safety of the vaccinations that all children are required to have before entering school. Concerns have been raised about the number of vaccines and whether we are overchallenging our children's immune systems. I understand that concern. But watch toddlers playing on the floor scooping up germ-laden objects and putting them into their mouths, and you'll see that they ingest bacteria, viruses, and foreign substances every day and, in doing so, activate their immune systems.

I also worry that we might be falsely led to believe that the deadly diseases of yesteryear no longer matter. If we stopped getting vaccinated in the United States, these diseases would become common once again, and society would be imperiled. From my travels overseas to third-world countries, I've seen the results of not getting "your shots." I've seen children with whooping cough in hospitals gasping for air, their chests moving as fast as they can, but still not being able to catch their breath. I've seen children paralyzed from polio, hobbling around on rudimentary handmade crutches. Millions of

TRUTH

After reassessing the safety of children's
cough and cold medicines, the U.S. Food
and Drug Administration says these drugs
should never be given to children under
the age of two. Why the warning? There
are a couple reasons. First, the dosage
margin of safety, even in medicines marketed to babies, is so narrow that these
preparations just aren't safe. They may
cause accidental overdosing and can interfere with the heart's electrical system,
leading to irregular heartbeats and
changes in blood pressure. It should go
without saying that it is never safe to give
adult cold preparations to children. It is always better to treat the specific problems
that a child has. That means narrowly targeted medicines for specific symptoms.
Mixtures are never a good way to go, even
for children older than age two.

people around the world are dying of diseases, including influenza, that are preventable and treatable with vaccines and other lifesaving interventions. It's horrendous and tragic. If vaccines were offered to those who do not have access to or can't afford them, outbreaks would be prevented in these countries and countless lives saved.

We tend to regard certain vaccines as a luxury because some shots are pricey and not covered by insurance. I can't argue that some are more expensive than others. But I can argue that the cost needs to be weighed against the cost of a human life. Remember that the vaccine for meningococcal meningitis, for example, at a mere eighty dollars, could save your child's life.

The same holds true for the human papillomavirus (HPV) vaccination that protects against cervical cancer. It is even more expensive — around $360. But compare that fee with the cost of cervical cancer, taking into consideration doctor visits, Pap smears, lab results, surgery, anesthesia, and perhaps radiation. There is no conceivable way that this cancer can be treated for $360. So doesn't it make sense to prevent the illness in the first place? It's this reasoning that led me to have both of my daughters vaccinated.

TRUTH

Doctors *do* want you to know about cures, natural or otherwise.

I get a little chapped when I read blurbs like "cures (or treatments) your doctor doesn't want you to know about" or "cancer treatments banned by the U.S. government." This is the stuff of conspiracy buffs. Being a doctor, I can tell you that we are, at our very core, healers. Why would we hide a cure or treatment for anything? Anytime there is a medical breakthrough, it is quickly announced and put to use — as the world has seen with antibiotics and vaccines. To suggest that the medical establishment would want to suppress or hide anything with the potential to heal is not only inaccurate but highly unethical.

HOW VACCINATIONS WORK

A vaccine works like this: Either a dead or a genetically altered or weakened (attenuated) version of the germ is injected into the body. The body recognizes it as a foreign protein and makes antibodies against it. When the "real" virus or bacteria invades the body, the immune system can identify the protein again, has the army to wipe it out, and can marshal a response before the disease has time to develop.

After you get a vaccination, it is not uncommon to have mild side effects. Most side effects are a little pain, tenderness, or even itching at the injection site. Sometimes you might feel achy or have a little fever. But that's about it. These are simple signs that you have a healthy immune system — and that it is activated and ready to go. It's your body's way of revving up its engines. Are there worse complications? Of course, but they are *very* rare. Every year, many, many more people die from infectious illnesses that could be prevented than from the vaccinations themselves.

Vaccinations are given on a set schedule, based on age groups and when we are at risk for certain infections. The reason for the schedule is that we know exactly when in life the body is exposed to certain germs and when it starts to make antibodies against those germs. Immunity from vaccines may not last a lifetime — we may outlive the initial protection of the vaccine — which is why you need "booster" shots, particularly after age thirty. Boosters serve as cues, or memory aids, to your immune system to remind it how to fight the germs for which you were originally vaccinated against. In many cases, boosters are suggested if you are traveling to a foreign country that is known to have large populations of unvaccinated people or recent epidemics. Plus, as we get older, our immune systems are not as strong. That's why influenza, in particular, can be so life-threatening to people in their eighties. There are other reasons adults need vaccinations: some of us were never vaccinated as children. If that fits you, talk to your doctor about catching up on your vaccines.

WHICH VACCINATIONS AND BOOSTERS DO ADULTS NEED?

The vaccinations you need depend on your age, health, lifestyle, and vaccination history.

Here's a rundown of some of the common vaccines you should get, based on recommendations from the CDC. You can get more information on adult vaccinations from the CDC website at www.cdc.gov.

Diphtheria, tetanus, and pertussis (DTP). This is a mandatory vaccine. All of us need protection from tetanus and diphtheria. Though best known for causing lockjaw, tetanus kills one patient in three, and diphtheria can lead to breathing problems, paralysis, and heart failure. Both diseases are now rare, thanks to childhood vaccination. Better known as whooping cough, pertussis is a highly contagious disease and one of the leading causes of vaccine-preventable deaths worldwide. Because the DTP vaccine provides only temporary immunity, err on the safe side by making sure you get boosters. If you didn't get these shots as a child, or you haven't had a booster in more than a decade, talk to your doctor about the vaccine. It's administered in a three-dose series, followed by a booster every ten years.

HPV (human papillomavirus). Approximately four thousand people a year lose their lives to cervical cancer, the second most common cancer among women. About three of every

TRUTH

You probably won't get much protection from the common cold by taking a daily supplemental dose of vitamin C, unless you run marathons, something I don't do because it makes me drop my ice-cream cone. This finding comes from researchers at Australian National University and the University of Helsinki, who reviewed thirty studies, conducted over several decades and included more than eleven thousand people who took daily doses of at least 2 grams — four times the dose normally found in supplements. Their analysis shows that vitamin C, also known as ascorbic acid, does little to prevent colds or reduce the length or severity of colds. However, they found that people exposed to periods of high stress — such as marathon runners, skiers, and soldiers on subarctic exercises — were 50 percent less likely to catch a cold if they took a daily dose of vitamin C. For the rest of us, please know that vitamin C can be harm-

Truth, *continued*

ful when taken in large doses over long periods of time. It can produce diarrhea, which can be dangerous in children and elderly people.

four cases of cervical cancer are thought to be caused by HPV, the most common sexually transmitted infection. Many of us are infected with this virus over the course of a lifetime but don't know it. Because HPV is a silent disease, women may be infected with certain strains that have been linked to the development of cancer.

There are now preventive vaccines that target the more virulent strains of HPV associated with the development of cervical cancer. The CDC recommends the HPV vaccine for all eleven- and twelve-year-old girls but allows for it to be given as early as age nine, long before they even think about being sexually active, so that the body can develop antibodies to the viruses. The vaccination is also recommended for women ages thirteen to twenty-six who have not been previously vaccinated or who have not completed the full series of shots.

The vaccines, however, are not perfect.

TRUTH

Most allergies are not dangerous, but some are. Anaphylaxis is the most severe allergic response (and thankfully the rarest). About 10 to 15 percent of the population may have an anaphylactic reaction to almost any allergen, including insect bites, pollens, some vaccines, medications, and certain foods. The reaction is almost instantaneous, and it is "systemic" (in other words, your whole system is affected). Symptoms include difficulty breathing because of the throat closing up, rapid pulse, hives or swelling, and in some cases, shock and cardiovascular collapse. Anaphylaxis should be treated quickly with an injection of epinephrine to open the airways. Normal antihistamines such as Benadryl can be taken, too, as soon as a reaction begins, but you do need to get to an emergency room pronto.

There are three shots, and all three must be given to fully protect a young woman. And the shots are expensive — as I mentioned, about $360 at the time of this writing. But, as is the case with so many breakthroughs, you can expect that the vaccinations will get simpler and cheaper over the next few years.

Unfortunately, one thing I don't believe you can expect is that HPV will go away in our lifetime. This vaccine is our best defense for preventing this sexually transmitted disease from causing cancer.

Measles, mumps, and rubella (MMR). This is another required vaccine. If you have not been vaccinated and have never had the infections as a child, or if you were born during or after 1957, you may need immunization against this trio of diseases, particularly if you do not have evidence of immunity — meaning you've never had the diseases or the vaccines. Health-care workers and women of childbearing age who are not currently pregnant may also need this vaccine. This vaccination is given in one or two doses, depending on your age.

Chicken pox (varicella). Immunization against chicken pox is usually given when you are a child. In other cases, people thir-

TRUTH

A food allergy is the result of the immune system's response to a particular food. When the immune system recognizes this food as foreign and a threat to the body, it goes into gear to do battle with what it thinks is the enemy. Milk, eggs, peanuts, nuts, soy, wheat, and fish are responsible for 95 percent of all actual food allergies. Eating a food you're allergic to causes the body to release massive amounts of chemicals, including histamine, for protection. It's the histamine that causes the symptoms of an allergy (which is why antihistamines work). A typical allergic reaction may include tingling in the mouth, swelling of the tongue and throat, difficulty breathing, hives, vomiting, gastrointestinal discomfort, drop in blood pressure, loss of consciousness, even death. Food allergies can be treated by avoiding the allergy-causing food or with a medication called epinephrine, used to control severe reactions.

Truth, *continued*

A food intolerance is just as it sounds. The food doesn't agree with your system. Lactose intolerance is the best example. People with this intolerance may lack a certain enzyme required to break down milk sugar (lactose), so when they eat certain dairy products, they may get diarrhea or an upset stomach. People with celiac disease cannot digest wheat protein. Other people have trouble with caffeine, chili peppers, horseradish, or hot sauce. As with food allergies, it is best to avoid the offending food or ingredient. A food intolerance is not usually life-threatening. Untreated celiac disease has terribly serious consequences, however: malnutrition, loss of calcium and bone density, and neurological problems. Someone with celiac disease who doesn't stick to the required diet can be at risk for several forms of cancer, including bowel cancer.

teen years of age and older (who have never had chicken pox or received the chicken pox vaccine) should be immunized. Adults who are not already immune to the chicken pox virus should also be immunized to protect themselves against this classic childhood disease. What's more, anyone over the age of sixty should get a booster shot. Chicken pox in adults is always serious. My sister did not have chicken pox as a child. Yet in her early forties, she contracted a full-blown case. There were blisters (pox) all over her body and even intravaginally. She had fever and aches and was out of work for two weeks. She was miserable, but it could have been worse. One adult patient in fifty develops complications such as brain swelling or varicella pneumonia. Health-care workers, women of childbearing age who are not currently pregnant, and those who live or work with children should also be vaccinated. A series of two shots is required for protection.

NEWS YOU CAN USE

Kill dust mites and other allergens in your laundry by washing it in hot water (140 degrees F). This is according to a study from the American Thoracic Society. Washing in hot water appears to annihilate 100 percent of dust mites, compared with only 6.5 percent when laundry is washed in 104-degree water.

If you haven't been vaccinated, get the shots. They're worth it.

Influenza (flu). Influenza is a serious respiratory illness — not just something that sidelines you for a few days with vomiting, diarrhea, fever, headache, or achy joints. It can be fatal, resulting in nearly thirty-six thousand deaths annually in the United States, according to the CDC. The recommendation now is for everyone to get a flu shot or the inhaled flu vaccine every year before the flu season starts. The vaccines work by exposing your immune system to the modified flu virus. Your body will then build up antibodies to the virus to protect you from getting the flu. The flu shot contains dead viruses while the nasal-spray vaccine contains live but weakened viruses — which is why you cannot contract the flu from either of these vaccines. The viruses in the vaccine change from year to year based on international surveillance and scientists' best guesses about which types and strains of viruses will be passed around in a given year. Some people who get the vaccine will still get the flu, but they will usually get a milder case than people who aren't vaccinated.

Hepatitis A. Hepatitis A is a viral infection

that is transmitted by eating food or fluids contaminated by fecal matter. This normally occurs when people don't wash their hands after preparing food, they have poor hygiene, or they are infected with the virus. People who use IV drugs are also at risk for catching hepatitis A. Fortunately, most cases are mild and do not cause permanent damage. But you will feel lousy with aches, fever, nausea, diarrhea, and sometimes jaundice. Severe cases can cause long-lasting liver damage. If you are traveling to undeveloped

TRUTH

"Stomach flu" is not technically the flu.

You've probably heard or used the term *stomach flu* to describe illnesses with nausea, vomiting, or diarrhea. These symptoms can be caused by many different viruses, bacteria, or even parasites. While these symptoms can sometimes be related to the flu, these problems are rarely the main symptoms of influenza. The flu is a respiratory disease, not a stomach or intestinal ailment.

countries and can't be sure about the safety of the food, this is an important vaccine to get.

Hepatitis B. This disease is transmitted by exposure to contaminated blood or semen. People who use IV drugs, those who have multiple sex partners, health-care workers, and in rare instances, people who have had multiple blood transfusions are at increased risk. While the symptoms may be similar to those for hepatitis A, the infection is far more serious. Long-term risks include chronic hepatitis, liver failure, liver cancer, and death. Most health-care workers are now required to get this vaccine, and it is routinely included as part of a child's immunization schedule. The vaccine, which consists of three separate injections, provides lasting protection. (As yet, there is no vaccination for hepatitis C, which is transmitted through sexual contact.)

Pneumococcal vaccine. Pneumococcus is a bacterium that often causes pneumonia, ear infections, and meningitis. It is particularly dangerous in people over the age of sixty-five and those with chronic health conditions. Like the flu vaccine, this shot is very safe and effective. One to two shots, depending on

TRUTH

Washing contact lenses with tap water can lead to serious eye infections.

If you wear contacts, you've probably been tempted to use tap water to clean them. How bad can it be? Well, plenty, it turns out. Besides damaging most lenses, this practice can cause serious eye infections. The results can be redness, pain, or blurred vision. And in serious cases, damaged corneas and even blindness. To avoid this, you should use a special lens cleaning liquid to wash your contacts and then immerse them in an overnight solution. And get in the habit of doing it every night, not just when you happen to think about it. Also remember to wash your hands before handling lenses. Every six months or so, you should get a new case for your contacts, sooner if it leaks. Finally, don't be afraid to break out that spare pair of glasses if you want to give your contacts, and your eyes, a break. A few days of rest won't hurt you or the lenses.

your age, will afford you protection.

Meningococcal vaccine. This vaccine protects against meningococcal meningitis. It is recommended for adolescents and should be mandatory for anyone living in cramped quarters like dormitories or military barracks.

Shingles vaccine. In May 2006 the U.S. Food and Drug Administration approved the first shingles vaccine, called Zostavax, for people age sixty and older. This is important, since shingles is a disease that primarily affects older people. Talk to anyone who has suffered through a case of shingles, and he or she will attest to just how terrible this infection can be. The shingles vaccine could make a huge difference as baby boomers reach their sixties, so if you find yourself hovering around this age group, talk to your doctor. A simple vaccine sure beats a couple of weeks of pain and misery.

Vaccines for travel. If you're planning on taking a trip to a foreign country, check the CDC website for vaccine recommendations, or visit a travel clinic in your area. Many foreign countries have very specific vaccine recommendations and won't let you enter unless you are properly protected. Plan ahead. Give yourself two months not only to allow your body time to build proper immunity, but because in some parts of the United States your doctor may not have the vaccine in stock and may need to order it. Be sure to keep an updated list of your vaccines with your passport and a second copy in a safe place.

Protect Others

The vaccinations I listed here are the ones I consider routine, and they will prevent you from most infectious diseases (other than the common cold). I also think being properly vaccinated is part of a bigger social responsibility, since vaccinations protect the people around you from getting sick and they protect society at large. One caveat: if you have cancer, kidney disease, or another chronic illness, be sure to check with your doctor to make sure your immune system is strong enough for the vaccine.

Keep Track of Your Immunizations

Regular adult vaccinations are vital. Stay up to date with your shots, and keep track of them. You can't always rely on your doctor to know which vaccinations you've had, especially if you've switched physicians over the years. I keep a file for myself, my husband,

and my kids, and it includes every shot they've had over the years. This information makes it easy when schools or camps want an immunization record. My personal record of immunizations is tucked away in a special form in the back of my passport, so that I know where it is at all times.

THE BRAVE NEW WORLD
OF VACCINATIONS

We are now in an exciting new era of vaccine research. The technology is being applied to far tougher challenges — such as using vaccines to attack the protein deposits that snarl the brains of Alzheimer's patients or even as a potential treatment for HIV or to fight off cancer or heart disease. Such vaccines are not like the measles shot you got as a kid, though. Take cancer vaccines as an example. Instead of inoculating a healthy person against a foreign body like a bacterium, these vaccines use proteins that are specific to the tumors. The vaccines trick the immune system into recognizing these proteins so that it then attacks enemy cells. Vaccines like this are already being used for the treatment of the deadly skin cancer melanoma, and the results are promising. In early clinical trials on people whose tumors had been surgically removed, those receiving the vaccine lived on average twice as long as control subjects. Vaccines against prostate, colon, and breast cancer may be on the horizon, too. In addition to using proteins from tumors, cancer researchers are also turning microbes into tiny Trojan horses that can sneak into tumor cells and destroy them from within. Anticancer vaccines are one of the most exciting areas of development in cancer research, and I believe that in the very near future there will be numerous vaccines against multiple cancers. Until then, the purpose and the promise of vaccines live on, allowing us to keep many life-threatening diseases at bay. Vaccinations remain one of medicine's greatest gifts to humanity.

■ ■ ■ ■

In the next chapter, I'll talk about something that's every bit as important as the annual checkup and vaccinations — how to get your doctor to listen to you, answer your questions, and treat you fairly and well.

MYTH #3 . . .

DOCTORS DON'T PLAY FAVORITES

Well, some do.

In a day I shall never forget, I arrived in the emergency room wearing the traditional uniform of a medical student — a short, white lab coat over my skirt. Like all med students, my pockets bulged like saddlebags with a stethoscope, charts, emergency room books, notes, pens, a flashlight, tongue blades, and other medical paraphernalia. It was like having your brain in your pocket, and I clinked when I walked. You could always distinguish a real "grown-up" doctor from us medical rookies because the attending physicians' coats were long and their pockets were empty, except for maybe a pen and a prescription pad. And, of course, the other distinguishing factor was my student name tag, identifying me simply as Nancy Snyderman, without the initials M.D. I hadn't yet earned them.

I was in my fourth and final year in medical school at the University of Nebraska in Omaha. As is typical in teaching hospitals, I had begun my "rotation" in emergency medicine, a required monthlong schedule that would give me an opportunity to evaluate emergency cases and present diagnoses to attending physicians — the fully experienced doctors on whose every word we hung. I was among a gaggle of med students who trailed these doctors around, entourage-style, like little ducklings, through curtains into examination rooms where they'd see patients.

ER doctors are a special breed. No other specialists in medicine treat the variety of conditions they do in a typical day. They patch up gunshot wounds, resuscitate patients, mend broken bones, open up blocked airways, bring down fevers, treat burns, stop pain, and combine all of this with hours of mundane stuff. Their work can require split-second decision making and rapid intervention before a situation spins out of control. Often, there is no real hand-holding, and most of all, there is no continuity. ER docs see cases through only snapshots of time — since patients are often whisked off to surgeons or other specialists for further care. Usually, as one of these doctors, you never know what the shift will bring or what will unfold. As a student, I was immediately drawn to those parts of it — the immediacy and the unpredictability.

That afternoon, a white woman who appeared to be in her midfifties came into our emergency room, unaccompanied. She caught my eye because her skin glistened with sweat, although the weather that day was temperate, not particularly hot or humid, and she seemed distraught. Probably a housewife from one of the many farms that dotted the landscape around Omaha, I thought to myself. She was full-bodied, with slightly graying hair that was styled in tightly permed curls framing her oval face. She could have been anyone's mother.

I noticed her for an unusual reason: unlike most ER patients, she didn't seem to be in any crisis. She was quiet. She wasn't bleeding, screaming, or struggling for breath. She had a purposeful steadiness in her walk, her jaw tight, as if she did not want to be distracted from the task at hand.

She registered with the unit clerk and was given paperwork to fill out. She retreated to a corner of the waiting room, settled on a blue vinyl chair, and scribbled in the required personal data. After signing the papers, she was asked to stay in the waiting room while the minutes ticked by.

Back then, we didn't "triage" in the emer-

TRUTH

It's true that the sooner you quit smoking, the sooner your body begins to forgive you. Within eight hours of quitting, the nicotine and carbon monoxide levels in your blood reduce by half, oxygen levels return to normal, and your circulation improves. In twenty-four hours carbon monoxide and nicotine are eliminated from your body, and in forty-eight hours the decline in lung function and excess risk of lung cancer halts. One year after quitting, your risk of a heart attack reduces by half compared with that of a smoker. After being smoke-free for fifteen years, your risk of a heart attack falls to the same as someone who has never smoked.

But unlike your heart or lungs, your colon is not so forgiving. Researchers have discovered that smoking creates a type of genetic damage known as microsatellite instability (MSI) that leads to colon cancer. MSI interferes with the ability of cells to repair damaged DNA, a process crucial to preventing damaged cells from turning cancerous. This research shows us that things we do can actually cause genetic changes in cells that may initiate a tumor. It is one more reason to stop smoking — and all the more reason to be watchful and conscientious about screening for this common cancer.

gency room the way we think of it now. (Derived from the French *trier,* meaning "to sort," triage developed from the need to prioritize the care of injured soldiers on the battlefield and later became an established practice in emergency rooms and trauma centers.) Basically, it means your condition is ranked, usually by a nurse, into one of three categories: immediately life-threatening, urgent but not immediately life-threatening, and less urgent. Triaging is necessary so that someone with a life-threatening condition is not kept waiting because they arrive later than someone with a more routine problem. The triage nurse records a patient's vital signs (temperature, pulse, respiratory rate, and blood pressure), then gets a brief history of the patient's cur-

TRUTH

Fortunately, there are many sources that can help with funding if you don't have the financial resources you need. The guide that follows will help you.

Community Health Center Locator

Find community health centers, migrant health centers, public-housing primary-care projects, and other sources of health care funded by the U.S. Department of Health and Human Services at www.ask.hrsa.gov/pc. You can search by location, types of program, and types of service. This information center provides publications, resources, and referrals on health-care services for low-income, uninsured individuals and those with special health-care needs.

The Eldercare Locator

The Eldercare Locator (toll-free at 800-677-1116) is a nationwide directory assistance service designed to assist older people and caregivers in finding local support resources for aging Americans to help them remain independent in their own homes. It provides names and phone numbers of organizations within a desired location, anywhere in the country, Monday through Friday, 9 A.M. to 8 P.M. eastern time. For TDD/TTY, access the relay service at 202-855-1234, or to reach a live operator, call 202-855-1000. The website is www.eldercare.gov.

Hill-Burton Free and Reduced Cost Care at Hospitals

Did you know that nursing homes and other facilities are required to provide a specific amount of free or below-cost health care to people unable to pay? Eligibility is based on the size of your family and your income. You can apply for Hill-Burton care at the facility where you were or will be treated. The website www.hrsa.gov/hillburton can help you find a Hill-Burton Obligated facility.

Insure Kids Now!

This national campaign links the nation's ten million uninsured children — from birth to age eighteen — to free and low-cost

Truth, *continued*

health insurance through the toll-free hot-line, 877-KIDS-NOW (877-543-7669), and a website, www.insurekidsnow.gov.

Medicaid

Medicaid pays for medical assistance for certain people and families with low incomes and resources. This program assists states in providing medical long-term-care assistance to people who meet certain eligibility criteria.

Medicare

The Social Security Administration and the HHS Centers for Medicare & Medicaid Services (CMS) are working together to provide people with limited income and resources extra help paying for their prescription drugs. The Medicare Prescription Drug Program offers help with prescription drug costs. The new program gives you a choice of prescription plans that offer various types of coverage. You may be able to get extra help to pay for the premiums, annual deductible, and copayments related to the Medicare Prescription Drug Program — an average of $2,100 in extra help.

The National Breast and Cervical Cancer Early Detection Program

Administered by the Centers for Disease Control and Prevention, this program helps low-income, uninsured, and underserved women gain access to lifesaving screening programs for early detection of breast and cervical cancers. The website, www.cdc.gov, can help you locate free or low-cost mammogram and Pap tests from your local breast and cervical cancer programs.

Pregnancy Care for the Disadvantaged

If you are pregnant but financially disadvantaged, programs in your state can help you have a healthy baby. They offer medical care, support and advice for pregnant women, and information about health insurance and other services you and your baby may need. For information on prenatal services in your community, call 800-311-BABY (800-311-2229). For information in Spanish, call 800-504-7081, or contact your state or local health department. The program's website is mchb.hrsa.gov/programs/womeninfants/prenatal.htm.

rent medical complaints and medical history to determine the appropriate triage slot. Even though emergency rooms didn't formally triage then, obviously if your arm was severed in a farming accident, you got in right away. But if your symptoms were nondescript, you'd have to wait your turn.

"Could you tell me what has been going on?" the attending ER doctor asked the woman, who looked pale and anxious. He listened as she explained her symptoms. She told him of experiencing vague chest discomfort and indigestion. No, the pain had not radiated down her arms, neck, or back. But it did feel like a knife going through her shoulder, she told him. And when she took a deep breath, she had the sensation of icy cold air that felt like it was singeing her lungs. No, she did not smoke. No, she did not have any heart disease in her family. She did not appear to be seriously ill and confessed that during her time in the waiting room she had begun to feel better.

The doctor listened intently with his stethoscope to her chest and palpated her abdomen — the basic perfunctory examination in order to arrive at a "differential diagnosis," a term for working backward from symptoms and creating a list of possible ailments to solve the patient's problem. He ordered an electrocardiogram (EKG), usually the first test given to someone who complains of chest discomfort. An EKG traces the electrical system of the heart and can sometimes show if a patient has had a heart attack. In a patient with a suspected heart attack, there is injured or scarred tissue, and the electrical activity measured by the EKG may be altered when it encounters this tissue. At the time it was the best diagnostic test we had. A chest X-ray, another common diagnostic test in these situations, was ordered to check for pneumonia, fluid in the lungs that can occur with heart disease, or even a tumor.

The results of both tests were normal. The doctor turned to his gaggle of young students and asked us, "What could this be?" We enthusiastically offered up any explanation that seemed to fit: gallbladder disease, an ulcer, dyspepsia. And then he quietly said, "She could be hysterical." He was referring to *hysteria,* a wastebasket term I've come to loathe. It is often used in a pejorative way to describe women who are upset. The word is derived from *hyster,* which means "womb" in Latin, and refers to a mental instability once thought to emanate from the uterus.

Everything appeared to look good. Feeling

better and given no better diagnosis, this woman was reassured that nothing serious was going on. She was given some antacids and an appointment to see a gastrointestinal expert the following week.

She walked out of the emergency room to her car and dropped dead in the parking lot.

In that instant, the scene began to unfold in slow motion.

I stood stock-still while I watched the ER team frantically try to revive her, half-expecting her to rise like Lazarus and come back from the dead. The rushing of doctors and nurses, the indignity of this woman lying on the pavement amid oil stains, a tube being thrust down her throat, the multiple attempts to shock her heart into beating again — it all morphed into the official routines of declaring the time of death and then assigning the task of who would track down, and call, the next of kin. I kept replaying the scene over and over again. How could this be? We just saw her.

Today, so many years later, ER physicians still miss the signs of heart attack in middle-aged women in 7 percent of cases, whereas male patients are misdiagnosed in 2 percent of cases, according to a 2000 study published in the *New England Journal of Medicine*. Even now, doctors fail to associate

TRUTH

Once dubbed a "vanishing practice" in the *New England Journal of Medicine,* the house call has made a comeback. Medicare data show a 37 percent increase to more than two million home visits by physicians from 1995 to 2005. Doctors who make house calls still carry a black bag — and it still holds a stethoscope — but it also contains high-tech items such as a cell phone and a personal digital assistant or laptop with patient histories, plus point-of-service diagnostic equipment, such as battery-powered electro-cardiogram (EKG) machines and portable lab kits. For information on physicians and other caregivers who make house calls, log on to the website of the American Academy of Home Care Physicians, www .aahcp.org. It lists a directory of doctors and other providers, like nurse practitioners and physician assistants, by state and zip code areas served.

heart disease with women. Mention the words *heart attack,* and even doctors are likely to conjure up images of a type A, stressed-out, middle-aged, and paunchy male suddenly keeling over at his desk. The statistics tell a different, startling story: heart attacks are the leading killer of women, claiming six times the number of lives lost to breast cancer. To this day, I believe that had a man come into our ER with the same symptoms that this female patient had, the ER doc would have pegged heart disease as the mostly likely diagnosis.

The details of her death — the scream for help from a passerby in the parking lot, the frantic exodus of doctors and nurses to the rescue, the defibrillation paddles shocking a lifeless body — left me with vivid images I will never get out of my head. This was my first, though not my last, encounter with what we now term *disparities,* or inequities, in health care. Disparities occur when members of certain population groups do not enjoy the same health status or receive the same level of treatment as other groups. Every day, for example, thousands of people in this country face difficulties in accessing quality health care or preventive services. Often the neediest, the elderly, women, and members of minority groups cannot get help

TRUTH

Technically, a preexisting condition is an illness you had prior to the effective date of your health insurance policy and is often grounds for denying insurance. But if an insurer rejects you, you do have some recourse.

- **Go insurance shopping.** Insurers vary in whether they will cover certain medical conditions. Some may reject you if you have diabetes; others may accept you if you control it through nutrition and medicine. Some insurers charge higher rates for certain medical conditions, so you have to do some homework. A good resource is eHealthInsurance .com, or call 800-977-8860 for information on which insurers might cover your condition.
- **Stick with COBRA.** This is a federal law that requires employers with twenty or more employees to let

them retain their coverage for up to eighteen months after they leave their jobs. You pay a higher premium than you did as an employee because you have to pay both the employer's and employee's share of the cost. But you can't be rejected or have to change your coverage because of your health.

- **Check out state high-risk pools.** More than thirty states have "high-risk pools," which must accept people with medical conditions who have been rejected elsewhere. And a few states, such as New York, New Jersey, and Massachusetts, are required to cover everyone regardless of their medical condition — a type of policy called guaranteed issue. There are downsides to high-risk pool coverage. For example, it is always more expensive than a regular individual policy, and there are waiting lists in some states to get into the pools. Ultimately, the cost of being uninsured can be far greater than the cost of your premiums. The rules and strategies vary greatly from state to state, but you can get a lot of information at your state insurance department website. Or go to the National Association of Health Underwriters' website (www.nahu .org). It can tell you if your state has a high-risk pool.

- **Fight back.** If an insurer rejects you, find out why. Often you can reverse the decision by providing additional information, including data from your doctor, or by clearing up any errors that might exist in your medical record.

and are disenfranchised from the health-care system altogether. So is a new class of the medically denied: the working poor — those who are in the workplace but make too much money to qualify for federal assistance, yet not enough to cover their own insurance premiums. These people fall through the cracks of the health-care system every day.

ANATOMY OF A MYTH
We know that disparities are widespread in

health care — thus myth #3 — because disease rates and survival rates among minorities and whites convey something less than a level playing field. African American men are 30 percent more likely to die of heart disease than non-Hispanic white males, for example, and Hispanics suffer in greater percentages than whites from overweight and obesity, two of the leading risk factors for heart disease. Cancer is the number one killer of Asian and Pacific Islanders in the United States. Prostate cancer strikes twice as many blacks as whites.

Many minority women do not have screening tests — such as Pap smears or mammograms — at their disposal. Because of this lack of access to screening, cancers are more likely to be in an advanced stage by the time they are diagnosed, which correlates to higher death rates from cervical and breast cancers.

Breast cancer, in particular, affects white women and women of color quite differently. White women are more likely to get breast cancer after the age of forty. In contrast, black women have a higher chance of getting breast cancer before the age of forty. Even more striking is the fact that black women are more likely to die from breast cancer at every age. They are 36 percent more likely to die from their cancer than white women.

As for other life-threatening diseases, African American, Hispanic, Native American, and Asian minorities are at a higher risk of developing diabetes than whites. HIV/AIDS, too, has had a devastating impact on minorities in the United States: racial and ethnic minorities account for nearly 68 percent of newly diagnosed cases.

Is there an easy explanation for why disparities exist? Yes and no. There are many reasons, often tightly knotted together and hard to unravel. Poverty, obviously, damns an ever-increasing number of Americans to substandard or nonexistent health care, but it is not the only factor. Education, family background, poor English proficiency, environment, diet, genetics, and other factors are at play, too. Even the biology of cancers may be different in black women, making the cancers more aggressive.

Another explanation is a lack of insurance. The number of Americans without health insurance rose from 41.1 million to 43.6 million from 2005 to 2006, according to a report released by the U.S. Centers for Disease Control and Prevention. There can be serious consequences when someone doesn't have health insurance. In one rather alarming study, uninsured women with breast cancer and men with colon cancer were twice as likely to die from these diseases as were insured people with the same illnesses.

Those with coverage usually have it through an HMO. HMO, of course, is an acronym for health maintenance organization, a form of managed care that makes choosing a doctor about as easy as choosing your parents. Some like to say it also stands for "help me out" — the desperate cry of people who are members of HMOs. Managed care works fine, as long as you stay healthy. The job of these companies is to regulate the flow of patients through the medical system while keeping costs down. You give up part of your paycheck for coverage, and all is well — until you become unwell. If you get sick, that's when things can get interesting. Remember, HMOs make money by keeping costs down. And that would be okay if it didn't mean denying you access to a specialist, a sophisticated test, or a procedure, which unfortunately happens all too frequently. Then you and your doctor may find yourselves arguing with a twenty-one-year-old HMO employee on the other end of the phone with no medical experience. Even for those of us who know this system, it can be arcane, confusing, and jeopardizing. And for

TRUTH

Until recently, men with osteoporosis have been underdiagnosed, inadequately treated, or ignored, even though two million American men have osteoporosis, and another twelve million are at risk for this disease. As a man, what can you do about this? For starters, teach yourself to trust yourself. If you have been taking certain medications for a long time, such as steroids, anticonvulsants, certain cancer treatments, and aluminum-containing antacids, or if you suffer from a chronic disease that affects the kidneys, lungs, stomach, and intestines and alters hormone levels, or if you engage in such lifestyle habits as smoking, excessive alcohol use, or lack of exercise, these are all major risk factors for osteoporosis. So are age and race (white men seem to have a higher risk). Taking your risk factors seriously is the first step to getting your doctor to take them seriously. Insist that your doctor pay attention and that the right

Truth, *continued*

tests be given. Doctors don't recommend that men supplement with calcium since this mineral creates risks for prostate issues. Guys: get your calcium from food.

another jolt, check the salaries of HMO executives and balance that with the health coverage you have been receiving.

Prejudice among health-care providers also produces deficiencies and indignities in the system. In 1999 a study published in the *New England Journal of Medicine* caught my eye. It demonstrated the impact of prejudice in deciding how to treat patients with chest pain. As part of the study, 720 doctors viewed eight videotaped patients — men and women wearing hospital gowns and staring at the camera. In reality, they were actors, four black and four white, who described identical symptoms of chest pain. Each doctor was asked to estimate the likelihood that a patient had a narrowing of the coronary arteries and then, based on the results of a stress test, to determine whether the patient should be referred to a cardiologist for a catheterization. This is a procedure in which a catheter is inserted into the heart via a

TRUTH

Sitting in hot water can have an effect on a man's ability to reproduce.

Thinking about becoming a dad? Then rethink relaxing in that hot tub. Sperm like cool temperatures to be healthy, plentiful, and motile, and the male anatomy is designed to accommodate this. Located behind the penis in a pouch of skin called the scrotum, the testicles produce sperm and testosterone. The testicles are located outside the body because sperm develop best at a temperature several degrees cooler than our internal body temperature. Water temperatures higher than 100 degrees F can affect spermatogenesis, or the process of sperm formation, and it can take up to six months to recover healthy sperm factors. These include sperm count, movement, shape, and structure — all needed for male fertility. So if you're planning on fathering a child in the near future, put off enjoying the hot tub until after your baby is born.

blood vessel in the groin. A dye is injected into the catheter, and as the dye mixes with blood it outlines the blood vessels of the heart. Images of the heart pumping blood through the vessels are projected onto monitors in a cardiac cath lab. By watching and guiding the catheter into the various blood vessels, injecting the dye, and studying the images, the doctor can assess how well the heart muscle is working and see whether there are any blockages in the vessels.

The results of this experiment were astonishing to me. The researchers found that women and blacks were 40 percent less likely to be referred for cardiac catheterization than whites and men. This means that doctors suspected heart disease 40 percent less often in women and people of color than in white men. What explained this outcome? The race and sex of the patient, whether consciously or not, played clear roles. Prejudice found its way into the exam room. There was no way around the results.

And heaven help you if you're overweight. Just recently, the *Journal of Clinical Oncology* reported that breast cancer patients who are either obese or poorly educated are more likely to get lower-than-optimal doses of chemotherapy — which could mean a failure to get adequate care. This treatment happens not only in cancer care but at many levels of society where people who are overweight or obese are often treated like second-class citizens. If you are struggling with your weight, there are many reasons for this, and no one should judge you for being overweight. You are who you are, not what you weigh. By the same token, try to examine your reasons for being overweight and attempt to get help — not because of societal pressure but for your health's sake. Never let anyone dismiss you or treat you unfairly because you have a weight problem.

I am equally worried by the indignities suffered by the elderly. Older patients are less likely than younger people to receive preventive care or to be tested or screened for diseases and other health problems. Furthermore they are consistently excluded from clinical trials, even though they are the largest users of prescription drugs. And our parents, our country's elderly, are quite deferential and polite when dealing with their doctors — which are not often qualities that open up the doors to good health care.

The sad thing is that health-care disparities are not going away, not in our lifetime nor in our children's. It doesn't take much imagination to realize that many of us could be on the list of people who are denied access to good health care. What can be done about all this? More than you think. If the system is not going to take care of you, then you need to know how to use the system. There *are* ways to get the most out of a medical system that isn't fair to women, minorities, the elderly, the economically disadvantaged, the uninsured, and others.

FIND DR. RIGHT

If we are to take care of ourselves, and live long healthy lives, we must know how to access the best health care, how to talk to doctors, and how to demand respect and appropriate treatment from a system that is not always kind to everyone in it. The first step is to select a doctor with whom you are comfortable. Patients, particularly minority patients, who have a regular doctor receive better care and have better outcomes if they get sick, according to a study by the Commonwealth Fund, a private foundation that supports independent research on health and social issues. They get the care they need. They keep up with routine screenings. They're better prepared to manage their chronic conditions. This study also showed that racial and ethnic disparities in access and quality are reduced or even eliminated when minorities have insurance and a "med-

TRUTH

Many people still think specific foods like chocolate, fried foods, or nuts will trigger pimples. This was roundly disproved decades ago by scientific studies showing that it is not diet but heredity and, to some extent, skin care that determines the predilection for this skin condition. The skin breaks out when pores get clogged with oils and bacteria. For many people, the condition is aggravated when hormones surge — during adolescence, pregnancy, and even menopause. You can't get acne, nor make it worse, by what you eat.

Acne can be alleviated by using medications that keep the pores open, control oil production, and eradicate bacteria in the skin. Look for topical products that contain salicylic acid. In extreme cases of acne, Accutane, an oral medication, can cure acne. But it is a serious medicine and is known to cause birth defects — which is why women who use this medication must abstain from sex or use birth control.

ical home" — defined as a health-care setting that provides patients with timely, well-organized care and enhanced access to providers.

Choosing a doctor is a very personal decision, and a vital one. Figure out what's important to you: Credentials? Personality — the right chemistry on which to build a long-term partnership? Bedside manner? Someone willing to explore alternatives? Someone who is older than you, of the same sex, or with a culturally similar background? Obviously, if you or someone you love does not speak English well, then your doctor of choice should be someone who speaks your native language, or you must take someone with you to medical appointments to interpret for you.

How are you treated? Behind your back, a doctor might call you "the gallbladder in room 310" or "the fracture in 420." That's just what we do and how we talk. You're more than just a gallbladder or a hip, and good doctors know that. So medical jargon aside, the question to ask yourself is, does this doctor treat me as a whole person? Life has taught me that spirit and body are one and that for most people the intimacy of first names and of a question or comment that reasserts a patient's essence and humanity, especially in times of trouble, is a part of healing. Look for a doctor who shows an interest in you beyond the specific physical symptoms he or she might be treating.

Know which hospital you would go to in an emergency and make sure your doctor has admitting privileges there. Does this hospital have a good reputation? One simple way to check a hospital's professional standing is to contact the regulatory commission that monitors health-care institutions, the Joint Commission for Accreditation of Healthcare Organizations (JCAHO) at www.joint commission.org.

Does the age, gender, or race of your doctor matter to you? Is your race or gender important to your doctor? Or are you looking for someone who is the absolute best in his or her specialty? My dermatologist is an African American physician whose practice is almost all people of color. Her office is very basic — no diplomas hanging anywhere — and there is often a wait. Some people might be put off by that atmosphere, but I go to her because she is highly competent, very smart, and a brilliant diagnostician.

Once you have found a doctor you like,

TRUTH

Bed rest isn't always best.

Used to be if you had a serious condition like recovery from a heart attack, your doc would want you to stay in bed for fear that activity might hurt or kill you. But now doctors want you up and around. And in the case of heart disease specifically, inactivity is dangerous. For other illnesses that require hospitalization, you'll be encouraged by your nurses and doctors to ease into physical activity, since extended bed rest poses risks for skin ulcers, pneumonia, calcium loss from bones, and deep vein thrombosis — the formation in veins of clots that can break free and travel to the lungs. We doctors now know that keeping people in bed can be bad for their health.

learn the rules and practices of your doctor's offices. Find out:

Who covers for your doctor when he or she is away or on weekends? Will you get the same level of care?

Does your doctor ever give out his or her cell or home phone number? And what is the best time to reach this doctor?

What insurance plans does the office take?

Do you have to wait long past your scheduled appointment time? Fifteen minutes or more without an explanation is unreasonable.

SPEAK UP AND STAND UP FOR YOURSELF

For most of us, standing up to our doctors, speaking our minds, and resolving conflict is really hard — even for those of us who are doctors. When we sit on that examining table as patients, the balance of power shifts. So it

NEWS YOU CAN USE

Want to get out of the hospital faster after having abdominal surgery? Chew gum. The bowel can stop working temporarily and be sluggish after the abdomen is surgically opened. It can be hard to eat and people can experience pain and vomiting. Chewing gum helps by stimulating nerves and hormones in the digestive system and can help you get better sooner.

is imperative that each of us speaks with a strong voice when it comes to our own health care. This is especially true for women.

Society conditions women to be well mannered and deferent when dealing with people; this serves us well in settings requiring etiquette and grace but not so well in medical situations, except for possibly getting a doctor's appointment earlier. You cannot afford to be passive or too accepting of a judgment or a test result you feel justified in questioning. You don't have to swap good manners for good care, but you do have to find your voice. And sometimes you simply must bully your way through hard situations.

Recently, I had a mammogram that for the first time in my breast screening history revealed an abnormal spot. When the mammogram technician asked me if I had time to get an ultrasound, I knew something was wrong and my heart started racing. I watched her draw a square around the questionable spot and try to figure out if the abnormal area looked like a cancer or not. I asked the technician if I could speak to the radiologist, who I knew was in the next room.

The technician was curt. "No, your mammogram results have to be sent to your doctor first. Then your doctor will go over your results."

This response really pushed my buttons. It was wrong and out of line. No patient should have to take that. I dug in my heels.

"Look, I am a doctor," I protested, "and that is not acceptable. I want to talk to the doctor today."

Why should anyone have to wait for four days for a radiologist to read a mammogram, then send the report circuitously to the doctor — especially when you already know that something is wrong? If, for some reason, the radiologist couldn't read the study on the spot, the technician could tell me that. I wouldn't let her dismiss me — and the problem — out of hand.

Refusing to budge worked. The radiologist appeared and clarified the findings for me. The abnormal area looked like a cyst and was probably nothing to worry about. This discussion took all of a few seconds. The technician wasted more time by fighting me than by just getting me help. There are times you must reach out and grab that starched white coat (figuratively, of course) and say, "I'm not done here; I have more questions." The assertive patient often gets the best treatment.

Try not to be apologetic in the aftermath

of dealing forthrightly with these issues. Women tend to feel guilty about being brash; we apologize profusely or write notes begging for forgiveness. We never hear of men doing that; they can argue, then unapologetically go out for beers together a few hours later. It's pretty clear that the spectrum of acceptable female behavior is narrower than the spectrum of acceptable behavior that men enjoy. But don't let that get in the way of your health. Bottom line: you don't owe anyone an apology for standing up for your medical rights.

BECOME MEDICALLY FLUENT

Currently, 45 percent of all U.S. adults, or 90 million Americans, can't read well enough to comprehend basic health information such as "take four tablets daily by mouth," according to a number of recent national studies. One of these, from Northwestern University, found that older people with poor reading skills had a 50 percent higher mortality rate over five years than people who could read adequately. Not being able to read well was the top predictor of mortality, after smoking.

The issue goes beyond the problem of poor reading skills, extends to people who do not speak English as a first language, and

TRUTH

Cracking your knuckles does not cause arthritis.

For years, I used to think that there was a connection between cracking your knuckles and getting gnarly, arthritic joints later in life. But I was wrong. Your knuckles are the bony protuberances of your joints that connect parts of your fingers to your hands. The joints are surrounded and lubricated by synovial fluid. When you crack your knuckles, you're pushing the joint out of its normal position. The bones pull apart, and the pressure on the synovial fluid is reduced. Bubbles form and quickly expand and then burst, hence the cracking or popping noise. If you make a habit of cracking your knuckles all the time, you may wear your joints down a little but not enough to cause arthritis.

spreads to other educated individuals who have a hard time comprehending medical advice from doctors. This "medical illiteracy" is a matter of life and death, and it affects people of all ages, races, income, and education levels. Understanding what your doctor is telling you during an appointment, or while giving a diagnosis, is crucial in terms of making the right treatment choice or following your doctor's orders. This is the person, after all, who will be explaining to you why you're sick, the tests you may need, the pros and cons of the various treatments, and why one option is being recommended over another.

Compounding the problem is that we doctors speak our own language — I call it doctorspeak — and it is rife with Greek and Latin. Learning that language is something we do in medical school. We unlearn words like "feel" because a real doctor will say "palpate." Likewise, we "auscultate" instead of just plain "listen to."

Every profession has its own lingo, and medicine is no exception. As premed students we learn the Greek and Latin roots of words, and as medical students we start incorporating them into everyday conversation — and we get comfortable with and proud of our language. We also speak in acronyms: bid, which is Latin for *bis en die,* or "twice a day," referring to how often to take a prescription medicine; it also means "brought in dead," which could happen if you don't take your pills *bid.* Then there is SOB, for *"shortness of breath,"* which is not usually a description of a patient's personality, unless of course the patient *is* an SOB. Another is UNIVAC, shorthand for "unusually nasty infection — vultures are circling." It also stands for Universal Automatic Computer, the world's first commercial computer that ushered in the computer age, making it impossible for anyone to do more than five minutes' worth of work without being interrupted by an e-mailed joke. NAD means "nothing abnormal detected"; if a superior asks for a test no one thought to order, in this case, it means "not actually done." We also use the letter *W* to signify someone's weight. To most, it is better known as a nickname for a GOP president known for his own skillful butchering of syntax and famous for uttering such quotes as "I just want you to know that, when we talk about war, we're really talking about peace."

Ever wonder where names for diseases come from? In the early days of modern medicine, a doctor would literally make a name for himself by attaching his name to a disease: Alzheimer's disease, Parkinson's disease, and Down syndrome, for example. These kinds of words are called eponyms. Eponyms are generally a good way to name diseases and medical conditions. For one thing, they do save time. Try saying "hyper-cortisolism from pituitary corticotrophin-(ACTH)-corticotroph tumors" three times in a row. On second thought, don't. Your doctor's visit will be over by the time you finish. Call it "Cushing's disease" instead.

Whether it is an eponym, an acronym, Latin, or Greek, doctorspeak affords access to an "in-group" language that connects all doctors to one another, from specialty to subspecialty, and to doctors around the world. It says "take me seriously" and commands respect when used among colleagues. However, when it becomes a part of our everyday language, especially when used in conversation with our patients, it is exclusionary. It puts up barriers instead of breaking them down.

Even if you did a lousy job at French or Spanish in high school, it's relatively simple to master doctorspeak. Mostly what you need to know are some simple prefixes, suffixes, and root words (which have their origins in Greek and Latin) and how they combine to form modern medical terminology. For instance, if you hear words ending in *ectomy* often enough, you can deduce that it's used to describe the surgical removal of an organ or body part. Your appendix is taken out by an appendectomy; swollen tonsils are cut out during a tonsillectomy. Take *hypoglycemia,* for example. Its word parts, all derived from ancient Greek, are *hypo,* meaning "under," or "deficient"; *glyco,* referring to sugar; and *emia,* referring to blood. When pieced together, the word *hypoglycemia* means "low blood sugar." Thousands of medical words have been constructed in the same manner. The chart cites other examples to build your medical literacy.

Doctors are trying to do a better job communicating to their patients, but they have a long way to go. A 2007 study published in the *Archives of Internal Medicine* found that doctors often talk about themselves too much in the first encounter with a patient, and patients don't like it because they feel it wastes their time. When a doctor can't connect emotionally with you, it's easy to feel alienated. Fortunately, many medical schools now offer sensitivity training. Several years ago, I participated in one such innovative course for first-year students at Duke University School of Medicine. Each student was given a card with a patient profile. Mine dictated that I play a wealthy widow with grown children; I had come to the hospital because of kidney problems. I knew I was better off than "patients" who were poor and alone, but even so, in the course of the

PREFIX/SUFFIX	EXAMPLE
Algia=pain	Neuralgia=nerve pain
Anti=attacks	Anti-inflammatory=attacks inflammation
Arth=joint	Arthritis=joint inflammation
Carcin=associated with cancer	Carcinoma=cancerous growth
Cardio=heart	Cardiology=study of the heart
Cepha=brain or head	Encephalitis=inflammation of the brain
Derm=skin	Dermatology=study of skin diseases
Dys=bad or abnormal	Dysplagia=abnormal cell growth
Ect=outer	Ectoderm=outer skin
Emia=in the blood	Toxemia=toxins in the blood
Endo=inside	Endoscopy=examining the inside
Gastro=stomach	Gastritis=stomach inflammation
Hemato=blood	Hematology=study of the blood
Hepat=liver	Hepatitis=inflammation of the liver

PREFIX/SUFFIX	EXAMPLE
Hyper=high, elevated	Hyperlipidemia=elevated lipids (cholesterol and triglycerides)
Hypo=low	Hypoglycemia=low blood sugar
Hyster=uterus	Hysterectomy=removal of the uterus
Itis=inflammation	Pancreatitis=inflammation of the pancreas
Mal=poor, bad	Malnutrition=poor nutrition
Myo=muscle	Myalgia=muscle pain
Necro=death	Necrosis=death of tissue
Nephro=kidney	Nephrology=study of the kidneys
Oma=tumor or cancer	Lymphoma=cancer of the lymph system
Osis=disease or abnormal condition	Arthrosis=abnormality of a joint
Osteo=bone	Osteopathy=bone disease
Ostomy=opening	Colostomy=an opening in your abdominal wall that is surgically created
Penia=loss	Osteopenia=bone loss
Trophy=growth	Hypertrophy=increase in the size of an organ

exercise I was either ignored or seriously patronized. When I protested some outrage, nurses would say things like "Isn't she cute?" I left the course with a profound humility that taught me how to better speak to my patients.

I don't think we can wait until our doctors get better at communicating. If you want the best medical care, you have to take charge. If your doctor says something you don't understand, insist that it be repeated in simpler language. Then repeat it back to your doctor to check your understanding. If your healthcare provider gives you a new device to use, make sure he or she demonstrates how to use it.

I'd like to emphasize one additional point: as a society, we Americans aren't comfortable talking about our own body parts. We consider it embarrassing or inappropriate. We use words like *private parts, down there, backside,* and other imprecise language, rather than describe sexual organs or specific areas of our anatomy. We even neglect to talk to our kids with the correct language, defaulting to words like "pee-pee" and "wee-wee" instead of penis and vagina. The trouble is, using fuzzy language is an obstacle to meaningful communication with your doctor. Telling your physician, "I have a pain in

TRUTH

Cotton swabs are for cleaning belly buttons, not ears.

Using a cotton swab can actually push earwax farther into your ear, impacting the wax and decreasing your hearing. There is also the danger of poking a hole in your eardrum, and that's dangerous. Like your oven, the ear canals are self-cleaning most of the time, and usually you never need to clean them. However, if you want to clean your ears, wash the external ear with a washcloth over a finger, but do not insert anything into your ear canal.

my backside" is vague. What does that mean? A backache? Or that it hurts when you poop? *Backside* or *down there* are not usually helpful answers. You've got to use the right words. Your private parts shouldn't be private, neither to you nor to your physician.

THE BEST REVENGE: LIVE BETTER AND ADD SEVEN YEARS TO YOUR LIFE

While we need to improve our imperfect health-care system, we also need to take advantage of what is right with it and not allow ourselves to make a lot of lame excuses for not taking care of ourselves. The best revenge against a system that is at times unfair is to be a healthy human being.

I was doing some research on this chapter — reading some of the literature published on disparities in health care — and I came across a fascinating study from Harvard University showing that you can add roughly seven extra years to your life by eliminating certain preventable risk factors and that doing so could be more important than access to medical care in terms of our longevity. What are those risk factors, that by doing away with, can help you live longer? Although some of these won't be a shock to you, take a look.

Risk Factor #1: Smoking. Quitting smoking can be tremendously difficult to do, and you may very well need help to do so — from your family and friends, your doctor, the use of a nicotine patch or gum, or a smoking-cessation support group. If you try but go back to smoking after quitting once, don't assume it's hopeless. The odds are actually better that you will quit for good if you have quit once or twice before.

NEWS YOU CAN USE

Not being able to get or maintain an erection (technically known as erectile dysfunction, or ED) definitely puts a damper on things. One way to avoid ED is to refrain from smoking. Cigarettes constrict the blood vessels in the body, including those in the heart and penis. Since blood flow to the penis is necessary for an erection, smoking may be the worst thing for your sex life. (Plus, kissing a smoker is yucky.)

Risk Factor #2: Heavy alcohol use. Curtail alcohol use, or don't use alcohol at all. More than one or two drinks a day can actually increase your risk of heart disease and cancer. It is hard on most organ systems of the body and can worsen your overall health when used chronically and to excess. You've heard that some alcohol is good for the heart, particularly red wine. That's true, in moderation. Moderation means that as long as you don't have a problem with alcohol, you may have one drink a day if you're a woman, two if you're a man. And if you find that your favorite alcoholic beverage is your next one, it might be a good idea to seek treatment.

Risk Factor #3: Overweight and obesity. Obesity is a risk factor for many diseases, including heart disease, cancer, and diabetes, and we know from other studies that it may shorten life span. The Harvard study advises maintaining a body mass index (BMI) of no greater than 21. BMI is a measure of weight relative to height and waist circumference.

Risk Factor #4: High blood pressure. Control high blood pressure. Reducing dietary fat and sodium works, as does exercise. But often these methods aren't enough, so you'll want to discuss medication with your doctor.

Risk Factor #5: High cholesterol. It's common knowledge that too much cholesterol

NEWS YOU CAN USE

Begin your meal with a low-calorie, broth-based soup. This may help you cut calories and ward off unwanted pounds, say nutrition experts at Pennsylvania State University. Participants in this study consumed 20 percent fewer calories when they started their meals with soup.

— a waxy chemical found in animal fat — is the scourge of a healthy heart. As I mentioned earlier, to help control my cholesterol, I was prescribed a cholesterol-lowering drug, but I was also told to make some dietary changes. I started thinking about how all the foods I liked would be bad for me. So out went everything with trans fats, those nasty substances that do to your arteries what bacon grease does to your sink drain. Then I threw out the beef, chicken, and cheese because they're loaded with saturated fats that raise your bad cholesterol level. Bad cholesterol is the kind that clogs your arteries, runs red lights, and violates parole. I started eating lots of vegetables. Vegetables on pasta, vegetables on rice, vegetables between slices of multigrain bread. I felt virtuous. But I'm not perfect. A few weekends ago I foraged through the pantry and found some chocolate candy bars in the back. I couldn't recall if chocolate raised cholesterol like saturated fats or trans fats do, so I ate a candy bar fast before I remembered.

Risk Factor #6: Not eating enough fruits and vegetables. Fruits and vegetables have more vitamins and nutrition than any other food, so whatever you can do — enjoying a salad

NEWS YOU CAN USE

Eating just one daily serving of whole grains can help lower high blood pressure, according to a study published in the *American Journal of Clinical Nutrition*. Examples of whole grains include corn, oats, popcorn, brown rice, whole rye, barley, buckwheat, and quinoa. The secret is to stay away from refined and processed breads.

a day, putting more veggies into soups and stews, or snacking on fruits — will greatly lower your risk for colon cancer, heart disease, and many other cancers, including esophagus, stomach, and breast. How much should you eat? The Harvard experts say at least 600 grams a day, or 3 or more cups.

Risk Factor #7: Inactivity. The Harvard study recommends exercising at least two to five hours a week, or what it would take to burn 4,000 extra calories a week — which is moderate, and that's something I like. You don't have to regard exercise as the equivalent of climbing Mount Everest, nor do you have to be fanatical about it.

Risk Factor #8: Illicit drug use. If you have a chemical dependency, you are not alone, and there are many places and ways to seek help. Begin by telling your doctor. He or she should be able to point you in the right direction. Seeking help for your problem does not mean you are weak. On the contrary, seeking help is a sign of strength.

Risk Factor #9: Unsafe sex. There was a time not too long ago when the only thing we thought of when we thought of safe sex was avoiding a pregnancy. Now it's not pregnancy we worry about so much, but our lives. I don't want to preach, but unprotected sex puts your life at risk. With any new relationship, you must use a condom and you should get a test for sexually transmitted diseases and HIV, too.

Bottom line: If you have any of these risk factors, take them seriously and treat them as an impetus to change your life. Keep in mind the possible payoff: seven years of healthy, vibrant living added to your life — as opposed to seven years on a ventilator.

ONE LAST THING

Hard as it may be to accept, there are grave inequities among the health care that we get. But you do not have to get burned by this

TRUTH

Approximately 19 percent of all women smoke, and though women are quitting daily, we are not quitting in the same numbers as men. One reason, according to the American Cancer Society, is that women are afraid to quit for fear of gaining weight. Women also have a more difficult time quitting, according to a study published several years ago in the *International Journal of Psychophysiology*. Women seem to be more addicted to the physical habit and sensation of smoke. Some studies show that the brain's pleasure centers in women excite when exposed to the smell or taste of cigarette smoke, while men require the nicotine hit to get the same response (which is why nicotine patches seem to work better for men than for women). Women smokers who do want to quit should try antismoking medications as one means to kick the habit.

ever-changing health-care scheme. All it takes is that you try to treat yourself well, and if you are in need of a lifestyle overhaul, change your life, little by little. Continue questioning what is good health for you. Ask the right questions, be sensitive to key issues in your personal health care, and be aware of where to go for help and further information. And you do need to be under the care of a doctor you like, someone whose medical judgment you trust. There are many health issues over which you have a lot more control than you think you have — and health disparities is one of them.

The next myth I'll explode is easy to fall for, and potentially deadly if you do. It's about a disease that is responsible for most of the deaths of men and women every year — but these deaths are largely preventable and I'll show you how.

MYTH #4 . . .

ONLY OLD PEOPLE GET HEART DISEASE AND STROKE

Maybe your older uncle once recuperated from bypass surgery after a major heart attack, or your grandmother suffered a stroke. Maybe you're someone who is always worrying about your elderly parent's blood pressure, cholesterol, diet, or lack of exercise — and nagging him or her to get checked routinely. You probably even know all the signs and symptoms of an impending heart attack or stroke, and catch your breath when the older folks in your life complain of a tingling arm, chest pain, or a sudden and surprising pain in the lower back.

But the fact is, you need to pay attention to all these factors yourself — no matter what your age. I imagine you're thinking right now, "Hold on. I'm only twenty. Give me a break." But guess what? The American Heart Association now recommends that young adults have a heart check beginning at the age of twenty, and every two years afterward. Why? For somebody who's heading for a heart attack in their forties, fifties, sixties, or seventies, there's arteriosclerosis building up in your teenage and young adult years. We are now seeing in children and adolescence the seeds of later heart disease. So if doctors start checking for basic things like waist measurement, blood pressure, cholesterol levels, body mass index (which is your weight versus your height), then preventive measures can be taken early on. Just because you are young doesn't mean you are at low risk.

The realization that heart disease could affect someone who was not older hit me personally a number of years ago. I had a friend, Mary, whom I had known since Girl Scouts, who had put weight on gradually over the years. Despite her extra thirty pounds, she was fairly active and liked to swim. One summer, when she was in her forties, she went for a dip in the lake, lost consciousness while swimming, and had a massive heart attack that took her life. There isn't a day that goes by that I don't think of Mary, and in the remembering, I have urged people I know to be as concerned about their own risk factors for heart disease and stroke — cholesterol, blood pressure, the fat content of their diets, smoking, and exercise regimen — as they are

TRUTH

Until recently, many cardiologists recommended supplementing with folic acid because this B vitamin seemed to decrease the risk of heart disease and stroke. Now they're singing a different tune. Folic acid is known to reduce levels of an amino acid, homocysteine, in the blood. A high homocysteine level, or hyperhomocysteinemia, has been implicated as a risk factor in cardiovascular disease. But new studies have proved that more folic acid is not better for decreasing risk. The American Heart Association does not consider hyperhomocysteinemia a major risk factor. Nor does the organization recommend widespread use of folic acid and B vitamin supplements to reduce the risk of heart disease and stroke. We all need 400 micrograms daily of folic acid, which we can get from eating leafy greens and some fruits and taking a general multivitamin. All women considering pregnancy should take a multivitamin that contains folic acid, not for cardiovascular disease but to protect against neural tube defects, a type of birth defect that includes spina bifida.

about those of an older relative.

Sometimes it takes a stricken celebrity to bring to light the truth about a disease. Not long ago, on the *Today* show, we did a story on Leean Hendrix, crowned Miss Arizona in 1998. At age twenty-six, she suffered a stroke and was taken to a hospital, where she was left lying in the hallway for six and a half hours, unattended, drifting in and out of consciousness. Because she was so young, doctors and nurses mistakenly assumed that she was either crazy or on drugs. She tried to explain that she was Miss Arizona and had never used drugs or alcohol. After an MRI, the doctors sent her home and told her to take aspirin, even though she was half paralyzed. The assumption by the medical personnel that she was doing drugs could have cost Leean her life. It shows, too, that the medical establishment is just as likely as a patient to agree on a myth without even questioning its validity. Leann's recovery spanned six months of intensive rehabilitation, followed by another twelve months of therapy. Today, Leann has no recall of her teenage years and has had to relearn math and how to drive a car.

ANATOMY OF A MYTH

I hear it all the time: "Heart disease, stroke — it can't happen to me. I'm too young." That heart disease and stroke are old people's diseases is one of the most insidious medical myths. Until recently, most studies on these diseases have been done on middle-aged men, promulgating this myth, but new studies prove that no age group is really immune. Still, this myth permeates the treatment of heart disease and stroke and ends up being translated into misguided reassurances such as "You'll be fine. You're too

NEWS YOU CAN USE

A good laugh is good for your heart. That's the word from researchers at the University of Maryland Medical Center. Watching a funny film may increase blood flow to the heart by up to 50 percent. Other medical experts say laughing a hundred times a day gives the same cardio results as working out for twenty minutes.

young to have heart disease." Sure, age is a risk factor, but it's vital to consider not just your age but other risk factors, too. High cholesterol, diabetes, high blood pressure, stress, lack of exercise, family history of heart disease, and obesity are all problems that can let you know you may be headed for trouble.

Heart disease and stroke remain the leading causes of cardiovascular disease and death in the United States. Although some heart disease can run in families, the majority of it has more to do with lifestyle and can thus be prevented and treated, either through diet and exercise, and sometimes with medicines. After I was diagnosed with a heart problem in my fifties (which I felt was too young), I realized I had done some harm in my youth when I was careless about what I ate. I'm glad I found out about this condition before it progressed, and now I'm taking action. I'm like a politician: I want four more years — and then some.

UNDERSTANDING HEART ATTACK AND STROKE

A heart attack happens when the flow of blood to the heart muscle is interrupted. Usually a clot lodges in one of the coronary arteries that lie on the surface of the heart

TRUTH

Your heart does not stop when you sneeze.

One of the myths surrounding a sneeze is that sneezing stops your heart. A sneeze is your nose's involuntary response to a nasal irritation or allergen. When you sneeze, you increase pressure within your chest and limit venous blood flow back to the heart. Your heart may make up for this by a slight change in its beating rate, but the heart and its electrical activity do not stop during a sneeze.

and supply blood to the heart muscle. Sometimes there is a prolonged spasm of one of the arteries. Think about it like a kink in your garden hose in which a little water gets through but not enough to water your lawn. That's the same situation here. A little blood gets through but not enough to nourish the heart muscle.

How can you tell if you're having a heart attack? The classic warning signs include pressure in the chest; radiating pain from the chest to the arms, shoulders, neck, or back and lower back; nausea; sweating; shortness of breath; dizziness; and fainting. Women's symptoms differ from a man's and include pain in the jaw; a feeling of breathing in icy air; pain or pressure in the chest, though it may not feel like a huge weight; or overwhelming exhaustion or fatigue. Radiating pain may not occur in women as often as it does in men.

A similar scenario occurs in the brain with a stroke. In fact, think of a stroke as a "brain attack." If one of the arteries in the brain is suddenly blocked by a clot, the surrounding brain tissue is deprived of oxygen. If an artery ruptures and floods the brain with blood, the surrounding tissue drowns and dies. Either situation can interfere with brain function and cause permanent damage. The warning signs of a stroke include sudden numbness or weakness in your face, arm, or leg, especially on one side of the body; sudden confusion; trouble speaking or understanding; sudden trouble seeing in one or both eyes; sudden trouble walking, dizziness, loss of balance or coordination; or a sudden severe headache with no known cause.

If people make healthy changes early in life, we find that we can prevent heart disease and stroke later in life — or, if you have the disease now, prevent it from progressing

TRUTH

Soft drinks may be linked to heart disease and diabetes.

Whether you call it "soda" or "pop," our love affair with soft drinks may be getting another reality check. Research now links soft drinks with increased risk factors for heart disease and diabetes. Researchers found that adults who drink one or more sodas a day — diet or regular — had about a 50 to 60 percent higher risk of metabolic syndrome, a cluster of risk factors such as excessive fat around the waist, low levels of "good" cholesterol, high blood pressure, and other symptoms. This news comes from the ongoing multi-generational heart study, the Framingham Study, which was begun in 1948 in a town outside of Boston. The latest findings included about six thousand middle-aged men and women who were observed over four years. They all started out healthy, with no risk factors for metabolic syndrome.

What is it about soft drinks that may alter your metabolism? For one thing, sweeteners, both artificial and natural, may increase the craving for more sweets, and people who indulge in sodas probably have less healthy diets overall. Another theory has to do with the colorings in sodas — particularly the caramel flavoring. It may interfere with insulin regulation, which also alters how well the body deals with calories. Diet or not, these beverages should be considered an occasional treat and not an everyday staple.

or even reverse it. So where and how do you begin protecting yourself? Start by knowing that heart disease and stroke are lousy conditions to suffer but that most cases can be prevented and/or treated — and easily monitored and screened for. This all begins with knowing your body on the inside as well as you know it on the outside.

KNOW YOUR BLOOD PRESSURE

When it comes to your blood pressure, knowing your numbers may be the simplest and most inexpensive way to get acquainted with what's going on inside your body. If you have high blood pressure, you probably do not know it, as high blood pressure does not

TRUTH

Eggs got a bad rap a couple of years ago because they have higher levels of cholesterol than other foods. Most of the cholesterol in eggs is concentrated in the yolk. But eating eggs isn't really how we get high cholesterol. When we eat foods high in fat, the liver turns some of that fat into cholesterol. There are a lot of other culprits in our food supply besides eggs that get turned into cholesterol, namely fatty meats and dairy products. Eggs are a great source of protein, and the white part is healthier and leaner than the yolk.

Like so many other things, enjoy your eggs in moderation. One egg contains about 213 milligrams of dietary cholesterol. According to the American Heart Association, the daily recommended cholesterol limit is less than 300 milligrams for people with normal LDL ("bad") cholesterol levels. So you can enjoy eggs several times a week, if you limit cholesterol from other sources — and skip the frying.

announce itself by exhibiting easily identifiable symptoms — which is why hypertension is often referred to as a silent killer. If hypertension goes untreated and undiagnosed for a long time, the nonstop pounding of your arteries under pressure speeds up the process of atherosclerosis. Untreated hypertension makes you a sitting duck for heart disease. The increased pressure in your arteries is like trying to force water through a narrow garden hose. The pressure will ultimately damage the vessel and it will leak.

Hypertension is also a major factor in strokes. The latest guidelines for blood pressure values are listed in the chart below.

Patients always ask me which number — upper or lower — is more important. Until recently, it was thought that the more important number in a blood pressure reading was the diastolic, or bottom, pressure. This is the

NEWS YOU CAN USE

Got high blood pressure? If you're overweight, modest weight loss — only 5 percent of your body weight — may be enough to bring your blood pressure down to normal.

pressure when the heart rests between beats. Systolic, or upper, blood pressure represents the pressure inside the arteries at the moment the heart is contracting. If you are older than age fifty, a systolic blood pressure of more than 140 is a much more important cardiovascular disease risk factor than diastolic, or lower, blood pressure.

I also explain to patients that there are basically two kinds of hypertension. Essential hypertension, which is the most common kind, refers to high blood pressure in which the cause cannot be readily determined. Secondary hypertension can be directly related to some other ailment, such as kidney disease.

If you have been diagnosed with high blood pressure, you will have to be vigilant in your daily life: be careful about the amount of fat in your diet (around 20 to 30 grams daily); ease up on salt; start exercising several times a week; stop smoking (the worst thing for your heart is cigarettes); and control your weight if you need to. If these methods don't seem to be enough, your doctor will want to discuss medication with you. Some of the commonly prescribed drugs for hypertension are angiotensin-converting enzyme (ACE) inhibitors, angiotensin receptor blockers (ARBs), beta-blockers, calcium

Pressure	Normal Blood Pressure	Prehyper-tension	Stage 1 Hyperten-sion	Stage 2 Hyperten-sion
Systolic (upper)	< 120	120–139	140–159	≥160
Diastolic (lower)	< 80	80–89	90–99	≥ 100

channel blockers, and diuretics. Many patients with high blood pressure require two or more antihypertensive medications to achieve their "goal" (optimal) blood pressure.

Today, there are simple kits you can buy in any drugstore that are easy enough to use at home. Ask your doctor or nurse to show you how to use it so that you can make sure the reading you get is reliable. Checking your blood pressure at home helps you keep it under control between doctor's appointments. It isn't an excuse for skipping appointments but rather an extra piece of information you give your doctor at your next appointment.

Home monitoring is important for another reason: if your blood pressure reading is high during a doctor's appointment, this could be "white-coat hypertension." It's worrisome, but shouldn't be. White-coat hypertension is

TRUTH

Dessert can be dinner.

Don't call the food police on me for this one, but I say you can enjoy a Rocky Road ice-cream dinner *now and then,* which means as an occasional deal and not a steady routine. Don't deny yourself certain cravings. If you make a meal out of a favorite treat from time to time, you'll be less tempted to overindulge on your splurge foods. This tactic can help you be more successful in controlling your weight over the long term.

a temporary rise in blood pressure caused by anxiety when a white-coated doctor or nurse enters the room. Anxiety causes blood pressure to rise, and going to the doctor makes many people anxious because they anticipate the worst. (Sometimes we don't wear white coats, but our presence can still evoke anxiety.) There is no way of getting around white-coat hypertension if you're susceptible to it. If you tell your doctor eating spicy foods gives you diarrhea, he will tell you to

TRUTH

My stubborn cholesterol level hadn't budged despite my best intentions. I pulled a friend of mine aside, Joy Bauer, who is the nutrition expert on the *Today* show, and asked her what I could be doing wrong. Her first question to me was "Do you drink unfiltered coffee?" I told her that I'm a coffee lover and have several cups a day, some of which I brew in my European-style coffeemaker that puts a little foam on top. She suggested that I start filtering my coffee — using paper filters rather than the gold ones — to see if this would help bring my cholesterol down.

This was a shocker to me. It turns out that filtering coffee with paper filters removes a natural compound called cafestol that can increase levels of artery-clogging LDL cholesterol in your blood. So now I sacrifice a little richness and save the strong unfiltered coffee like espresso, cappuccino, Turkish coffee, and coffee

Truth, *continued*

brewed from those French press cof-
feemakers for an occasional treat. And
yes, my cholesterol came down.

stop eating spicy foods. But if you tell him
doctor's visits give you high blood pressure,
he will never tell you to stop going to the
doctor. Once you go home, your blood pressure will usually return to normal, and you
can confirm this by home monitoring.

KNOW YOUR LAB NUMBERS

Heart disease and stroke can be prevented
most effectively if you go on the offensive
with laboratory tests, performed by drawing
several tubes of blood. Don't worry about
how much blood is drawn; your body goes to
work right away at making more. There are
trusted indicators that are invariably accurate in predicting risk, in addition to blood
pressure, and these include elevated triglyceride and cholesterol levels. Also important
are creatinine, potassium, platelets, and glucose. Learning what your lab numbers mean
can help you exert greater control over your
cardiovascular health. Healthy targets for
these numbers have dropped, or have been

modified, in recent years, so it's worth a brief review.

Total cholesterol. This is the number that most of us remember. A total cholesterol

---

TRUTH

Having sex after a heart attack is just fine.

As soon as you are able to walk up two flights of stairs without severe shortness of breath, feeling light-headed, or feeling your heart skip, it is generally assumed that you are ready to resume the enjoyment of sex. This usually (but not always) occurs within a month of a heart attack. As with all areas of your life, use common sense. Just as you would not resume driving alone immediately, without the aid of another driver, you will want to go slowly in the bedroom. Talk to your partner, stop and rest if you need to, try again, talk about it again, build back the connection, step by step. And if your lovemaking depended on advanced calisthenics, you may have to modify your approach slightly.

---

reading that is lower than 200 milligrams per deciliter of blood (mg/dL) is considered healthy; a reading higher than 200 mg/dL can raise the threat of heart disease. Your doctor, however, is more likely to pay attention to other, more revealing numbers, particularly LDL, low-density cholesterol, the bad kind that causes arterial plaque.

LDL cholesterol. The newest findings indicate that LDLs below 130 mg/dL are ideal; below 100 mg/dL, if you are already at risk for heart disease, with two or more risk factors like high cholesterol, high blood pressure, overweight, or a family history; and below 70 mg/dL, if you are at extremely high risk (you smoke, have diabetes, have high blood pressure, or have suffered at least one heart attack). There are dietary moves you can make against high LDL: increasing fiber in your diet, cutting back on saturated fat, and eating more fruits and vegetables. If taking all these steps does not make a difference, your doctor's next line of defense will probably involve drug therapy: statins, effective medications that inhibit the production of cholesterol in your liver, or other LDL-taming drugs such as bile acid sequestrants and fibric acids.

TRUTH

The life you save may be your own. Preliminary studies suggest you can lower your risk of heart disease by regularly giving blood. This helps mitigate the amount of iron in your body. Many researchers think that we take in too much iron, mostly from eating red meat. Excess iron is thought to aid in the creation of free radicals in the body, speeding the aging process and raising the risk of heart disease, cancer, and Alzheimer's disease. Until menopause, women are naturally protected from iron overload, but after that the danger of overdose climbs. But don't rely on donating blood alone. Go easy on the red meat: no more than a few servings a week and keep each to the size of a deck of cards.

HDL cholesterol. High-density lipoprotein, or HDL, may actually help in preventing atherosclerosis. With this number, the higher the better. Ideally, you will want to have an

HDL level above 60 mg/dL; lower than 40 mg/dL is a red flag for potential problems. Losing weight, exercising, smoking cessation, eliminating trans fats, eating more fiber, and increasing your intake of monounsaturated fats like olive or canola oil can help

TRUTH

Thin people die of heart attacks every day.

Just because your weight is normal doesn't mean you are out of the woods when it comes to heart disease. Knowing the health of your blood and your heart is just as important as knowing your weight. Some people are born with a genetic predisposition to high cholesterol. They may look like the picture of health from the outside, but inside they can have dangerous plaque blocking their coronary arteries, the arteries that surround the heart. Know your total cholesterol, the breakdown of the "good" and "bad" components of cholesterol, and your triglycerides. And don't smoke. Smoking is the fastest way to a heart attack.

hike your HDL cholesterol. One of the most effective drugs for raising HDL levels is a prescription form of the B vitamin niacin, called Niaspan.

Triglycerides. A fat in the body and the blood, triglycerides are generally considered normal at levels less than 150 mg/dL. If you have a high triglyceride level, you will want to lower that through diet (limiting processed foods and sugars), weight loss, and exercise.

Creatinine. This is a muscle-breakdown product, which, like household garbage, gets ousted from the body by the kidneys at a steady rate. A buildup of creatinine in the body can be a sign that the kidneys aren't working well, and kidney dysfunction is a strong risk factor for heart disease and stroke. If your kidneys are healthy, your creatinine levels will be about 1.3 mg/dL or lower. Creatinine is measured from a routine test called a comprehensive metabolic panel, frequently ordered at your annual physical.

Platelet (thrombocyte) count. Tested through a routine complete blood count test, platelets (thrombocytes) are the smallest type of blood cell and play a major role in

TRUTH

People with diabetes can eat sweets or chocolate.

Before doctors were able to closely monitor patients and regulate blood sugar better, people with diabetes were told to absolutely avoid certain foods. Teenagers, forbidden to eat cake, were cut off from birthday parties and other celebrations for fear that they might have a diabetic crisis. Food became the enemy rather than an essential part of a diabetic's life. According to the American Diabetes Association, you can enjoy sweets and desserts in moderation if eaten as part of a healthy meal plan or when combined with exercise. These foods are no more off limits to people with diabetes than they are to non-diabetics.

blood clotting. If there are too few platelets, uncontrolled bleeding may be a problem. If there are too many platelets, there is a risk of a blood clot forming in a blood vessel. Also, platelets may be involved in atherosclerosis. A normal platelet count is about 150,000 to

450,000 platelets per microliter of blood.

Potassium. Doctors look at levels of this common blood salt to see whether you can take certain blood pressure medications commonly prescribed to people with cardiac risk factors like high blood pressure. Normal potassium levels range from 3.5 to 5.0 mil-

---

TRUTH

Body build can indicate an increased risk of heart disease.

Think apple and pear. Knowing which fruit best describes your body may help you understand your predilection for heart disease. If you tend to put on weight in the upper body or in the stomach or midsection, you are an apple. The fat you see on the outside is also on the inside, wrapping its way around your organs. This is toxic fat that is linked to diabetes and heart disease. If you carry most of your weight on your hips, you are probably pear shaped. This fat is not as dangerous. It can be just as tough to take off, but there isn't as strong a link to cardiovascular disease.

TRUTH

Breathing in secondhand smoke is like sucking on the exhaust pipe of a city bus. The smoke that comes out of the end of a cigarette and out of someone's mouth is loaded with toxins and carcinogens that are known to cause cancer. Secondhand smoke takes fifty thousand lives every year, and women and children are particularly susceptible. For example, women who don't smoke but live or work with people who do have a 27 percent increased risk of breast cancer and are twice as likely to develop cervical cancer. Other studies clearly connect secondhand smoke to an increased risk of lung cancer, lung disease, and heart disease.

Another form of secondhand smoke you might not be aware of can occur when you nurse your infant. That's right. As a new mom, if you smoke before breast-feeding, your baby will sleep less and not as well and wake up from naps sooner, according to a 2007 study published in *Pediatrics*.

The nicotine in cigarettes is passed to infants through breast milk and alters a baby's sleep patterns.

Exposure to secondhand smoke is a health-destroying, life-threatening issue — and one reason why public buildings should ban smoking at entryways. We are all entitled to clean air.

limoles per liter (mmol/L). Potassium testing, along with other electrolytes, is frequently ordered as a part of a routine annual physical.

Glucose. The standards for glucose, or blood sugar, have changed in recent years. Levels below 100 mg/dL are normal. If your numbers after fasting are above 126, you might have diabetes, a risk factor for cardiovascular disease. Levels between 100 and 125 may indicate "prediabetes," a condition that is largely reversible with attention to nutrition, weight control, exercise, and sometimes oral diabetes medication.

Take an interest in these numbers, and you can make a real difference in the outcome of your health and any treatment your doctor

TRUTH

Experts think being a couch potato accounts for more illness and death than anything except for cigarette smoking. I was startled to find out that no less than 49 percent of all Americans do practically nothing to keep fit. This isn't good, and we have to change it. Just recently, brand-new guidelines were issued on exactly how much exercise the human body needs. The old guidelines, crafted in 1995 by the American College of Sports Medicine (ACSM) and the U.S. Centers for Disease Control and Prevention, said: "Every U.S. adult should accumulate 30 minutes or more of moderate-intensity physical activity on most, preferably all, days of the week." The new guidelines, put together by the ACSM and the American Heart Association, call for healthy adults to engage in moderate-intensity aerobic physical activity for at least thirty minutes five days each week, such as a brisk walk or light jogging, or vigorous-intensity aerobic exercise like jogging or running for at least twenty minutes three days a week. The guidelines also recommend weight training to work on muscular strength and endurance, with eight to ten different exercises on two nonconsecutive days a week. An easy way to get yourself moving is to log ten thousand steps a day. That's the equivalent of five miles and burns anywhere from 400 to 500 calories a day. To get started, wear a pedometer for a few days while going about your normal day to see how many steps you ordinarily take. Then add about one thousand steps (half a mile) each week, building up to ten thousand steps or more a day. Studies so far show that taking ten thousand steps or more a day stimulates weight loss and reduces blood pressure.

recommends. If you find that any of your numbers are out of the normal range, you can turn a negative into a positive with the right lifestyle changes.

CONSIDER ASPIRIN THERAPY

When used to complement a preventive health program, aspirin guards against heart

TRUTH

While fats all have the same number of calories, they don't all act the same way inside your body. Some fats are better for you than others. Fish oil, for example, is the best fat around. It protects against stroke and heart disease, it is good for your brain, and it has a positive effect on your inflammatory response. But unlike some other fats, this isn't one you can drizzle over your salad or cook with. Still, you can eat the real thing by having fish three to four times a week. If you can't eat that much fish, supplement your diet with fish oil capsules. If you need a good oil for cooking, stick with olive oil or canola oil. Both are high in monounsaturated fats. Why does that matter? Because eating them sparingly helps reduce the risk of coronary heart disease by keeping LDL cholesterol (the "bad" kind) in check.

TRUTH

I have a very good friend who is a famous surgeon. No one would ever say that she is skinny — never. But she is one of the fittest women I have ever known and could run me under the table. She is the best example I know that being skinny is not the same as being fit. Now research proves it. A large study of women with heart problems, the Women's Ischemia Syndrome Evaluation, found that active women, no matter how thin or fat, were much less likely to have a heart attack or other cardiac problems than women who didn't exercise. Don't mistake the message: this is not a license to pack on pounds. Other large-scale studies have shown that being overweight or obese, regardless of how much we exercise, does spike our risk of diabetes. The bottom line is to move, stay in shape, and think like an athlete.

TRUTH

Men don't like to dial 911.

Calling 911 and asking for directions have something in common. Men, apparently, don't like to do either, according to a recent Minnesota study of 1,263 patients who suffered a major heart attack. Researchers found that 37 percent of men from rural communities were rushed to a hospital in an ambulance, compared with 49 percent of rural women. The rest of both sexes drove themselves or were taken by a friend or family member.

The most successful treatment for a heart attack is immediate and aggressive. Don't be afraid to call 911. The goal is to get to the hospital as soon as possible, without aggravating the situation and before permanent damage to the heart muscle has been done.

disease, curbs heart attacks, protects colon health, and more — in addition to its main job as a painkiller. A lot of doctors are afraid to say, "Go on it," but aspirin is clearly a life-

TRUTH

There's an old lament that goes like this: "God, if I can't be skinny, please make all my friends fat." But be careful what you wish or pray for. Research from Harvard Medical School says that obesity can be socially contagious; in other words, having fat friends or family around can make you fat. For example, if your close friend becomes obese, your chances of becoming obese increase 57 percent; if your siblings are fat, the increase is 40 percent; and if your spouse is hefty, the increase is 37 percent. One explanation is that friends affect one another's perception of fatness. When a close friend becomes obese, being fat may not look so bad. We're also influenced by other people's eating habits: when everyone around us is eating, we join right in. If you're overweight, take charge of your health, especially since studies report that being obese can reduce your life span by 22 percent (that's about thirteen years). Spend time with

Truth, *continued*

obese friends at events that don't involve food. Join a gym where you can make new, fitness-minded connections. And join a weight-loss support group for extra encouragement.

saver. I tell my patients that if aspirin were new and presented to the U.S. Food and Drug Administration for approval today, approval would be held up for years because of the drug's many uses and certain of its side effects. And, if it finally did pass, aspirin would probably cost a dollar a pill!

On pharmacy shelves are both generic and brand-name aspirin. I prefer the generic variety, the kind that most people don't think is as good because it is powdery and tends to fall apart. However, that's exactly what you want because it dissolves so easily in your gut.

Aspirin is available in only two different doses: regular, which is 325 milligrams per pill, and low dose, formerly called baby aspirin, which is 81 milligrams per pill. There's no such thing as a "baby aspirin" anymore. No aspirin is safe for kids or teens, since it's been linked to a fatal condition called Reye's syndrome.

Important considerations about aspirin are when to take it and to discuss its use with your physician. The American Heart Association recommends a low-dose aspirin a day for:

- Women over age sixty-five (if the benefits outweigh the risks)
- Men over age forty-five, to prevent heart attack

If you think you're having a heart attack, chew an aspirin immediately — any dose will do — and then head to the hospital. As an anticlotting agent, aspirin works by preventing platelets, tiny clotting elements in the blood, from clumping together, thus busting a clot. Within fifteen to twenty minutes of chewing that aspirin, it will start to dissolve a clot, and that's precious time.

The Aspirin Foundation recommends aspirin therapy during a current cardiovascular event (for example, taking a tablet of aspirin if you're experiencing chest pain probably due to a heart attack); if you're at risk of a heart attack but haven't yet had one; and if you've had a heart attack and want to reduce the risk of a second one. Of course, don't start aspirin therapy unless your doctor okays it.

Do not reach for the aspirin bottle if you think you are having a stroke, however. In some strokes, an area of the brain is flooded with blood, and taking aspirin could intensify the bleeding. You don't know what kind of stroke you're having until you're evaluated, so hold off on taking anything until you're seen by a physician in the emergency room.

As amazing as this drug is, it is not for everyone, particularly those with ulcers, especially bleeding ulcers, and no one 18 or younger should be given aspirin. Keep in mind that aspirin is still a medicine with side effects, such as stomach bleeding. Aspirin can thin your blood, too, making you bruise or bleed more easily should you injure or cut yourself.

NO MORE STROKES!

Fatty deposits caused by atherosclerosis can clog the carotid and vertebral arteries that carry blood from the heart to the brain, and if these blockages go untreated they can cause a stroke. If your doctor believes you're at risk for vascular disease, he or she may recommend a test that shows how blood is flowing through the vessels. One of the easiest tests is an ultrasound, and with these

TRUTH

Fat-free foods can wreck your diet.

Just because the label professes "fat-free" or "reduced fat" doesn't guarantee calorie-free. Some diet products like sugar-free cookies or ice cream, fat-free ice-cream toppings, and reduced-fat peanut butter have become hot items, but they can contain just as many calories at their regular counterparts, which means they're just as likely to promote weight gain. You can do the comparisons yourself by reading nutritional labels and comparing the calorie counts among foods. The labels are consistent, and once you get used to reading them, you'll find it unbelievably easy. One caveat: make sure you notice how many "servings" are in each container (there may be multiple servings), or you could be in for a real calorie shock.

sound waves any narrowing of the arteries in the neck is easy to see (interesting, isn't it, that we can see through sound?). Should your doctor be concerned about a blockage located high in the neck or in the brain, he or she may order an MRI or an angiogram. Both tests are good, but there is nothing better than never needing them. The biggest secrets for getting out of these tests are also the most boring. We all know that we should eat healthy foods, exercise on a routine basis, and not smoke. But that's only the beginning. Sometimes we might have to take medication and watch other aspects of our lifestyle. Heavy drinking, for example, raises the risk of stroke and high blood pressure, too. Although a certain amount of alcohol may help prevent cardiovascular disease, more than one or two drinks a day is health-risky.

This leads to a discussion of atrial fibrillation (AF), a condition in which the upper chambers (atria) of the heart beat irregularly. This alters how efficiently blood is pumped through the atria and the ventricles (the two lower chambers of the heart) and out to the body. AF results in the blood pooling in these chambers. Because the blood is being pushed through forcefully and settling into little puddles, it may clot. Any clot can break loose and end up in another part of the body. If it travels to your brain, you end up having a stroke. In fact, AF is the leading cause of stroke, so you'll want to find out if

TRUTH

Type 2 diabetes is just as serious as type 1 diabetes.

Diabetes is a condition that causes you to have too much sugar in your blood. In type 1 diabetes, for example, the pancreas is not able to produce or isn't producing enough insulin — the hormone that helps your blood assimilate sugar and turns the sugar into fuel. People with type 1 diabetes need supplemental insulin daily for survival. In type 2 diabetes, the body makes insulin, but the cells have trouble using it. You may have heard that this type of diabetes is not as serious as type 1. Not true! Both types of diabetes put you at a higher-than-average risk for heart attack, stroke, kidney disease, and other serious complications.

you have it. Your doctor will likely check your pulse to see if it is strong and regular. An EKG is the best way to check the electrical system in the heart and can show if the atria and ventricles are working together. Your doctor may also suggest that you wear a heart monitor for twenty-four hours. This is like wearing a purse over your shoulder that is attached to electrodes on your chest. If there is a problem, this kind of monitoring will pick it up. The good news is that AF can be controlled through drug therapy, usually with blood thinners like aspirin or warfarin (Coumadin), or medications used to slow down the rapid heart rate associated with AF, such as digoxin, beta-blockers, calcium antagonists, and others. If medications fail, this condition can be treated through the insertion of a pacemaker or miniature defibrillator. Treating AF is an important way to help prevent stroke.

I want to reassure you: not all irregular heartbeats indicate AF. Most irregular heartbeats (arrhythmias) are benign, and everyone has them now and then. It's easy to get worried about them because we can feel them as they're happening, and after all, this is your heart. The heart, though, is perhaps the toughest and most reliable organ in your body. It goes all day and all night, pumping blood, taking the abuse of a few extra pounds or the occasional cigarette. An infrequent skip, quiver, or extra beat doesn't mean your heart is going to stop. Irregular heartbeats can have a variety of triggers — stress, too much caffeine, excess alcohol or other drugs, smoking, anxiety, or medications. Any irregular heartbeat needs to be evaluated in light of everything else that is going on in your life, including any symptoms of existing heart disease. But don't hesitate to call your doctor if a heart rhythm irregularity is accompanied by a rapid thumping or pounding sensation in your chest, chest discomfort, fatigue or lightheadedness, fainting, or shortness of breath.

RECOGNIZE TIAS

Growing up in Fort Wayne, Indiana, I loved listening to the adventures of my maternal grandfather, who once worked on the Union-Pacific Railroad as a young man and still remembered train schedules down to the minute. One afternoon, as I sat captivated by his stories of hoboes who would hitch rides across the Missouri plains, I noticed that his words were slurred, or dropped altogether, and didn't make sense. He seemed to lose his place in the story. At first I thought it was grandfather silliness, but then I got scared and confused. But no sooner had I noticed something wrong than he was back on track, picking up where he left off. Now I know that my grandfather was having a classic transient ischemic at-

215

tack, or TIA.

A TIA is a ministroke. Its symptoms are similar to those of a stroke but with two very important exceptions: they are transient, gone within five minutes, and there is no permanent damage. TIA is most often the result of atherosclerosis, but it may also occur if you have high blood pressure, if you smoke, or if you have diabetes. TIA should be considered a warning sign that a stroke may be looming. Of people who've had one or more TIAs, more than a third will later have a stroke. If you have suffered a TIA, discuss with your doctor ways to minimize the possibility of a future stroke. Depending on your symptoms and the problems your doctor may suspect you have, there are a variety of tests available — generally the same tests used to diagnose stroke: imaging tests like CT scans or MRIs to give a picture of the brain; electrical tests that record the electrical impulses of the brain; and blood flow tests like ultrasound or angiogram, which give a picture of the blood flow through the vessels. If there is a blockage, it can be treated with medicine or surgery. If your arteries look clear, your doctor may recommend aspirin or a blood thinner to keep the blood from clotting too readily.

TRUTH

The word from Harvard researchers is that there are seven counties in the United States, all found in the Centennial State, that have the greatest average life expectancy. (Those counties are Clear Creek, Eagle, Gilpin, Grand, Jackson, Park, and Summit in case you're thinking about loading up a moving van.) The study doesn't pinpoint what's so special about Colorado; perhaps the longevity of its residents has something to do with cleaner air and the mountainous terrain, which makes it easy to be active and keep the body moving.

GIVE YOUR FAMILY THE GIFT OF GOOD HEALTH

With heart disease and stroke now affecting the very young, prevention has to be a family affair. Even if you are not conscious of it, your kids will take cues from you — everything from how you eat to whether you exercise, so you'll want to pay attention to the

217

habits you model.

Take a look around your kitchen, and you'll likely find more meats and snack foods than fruits and vegetables. Yet there's ample evidence showing that ten servings a day of the latter (before you balk, that's not as much as you think: one serving is equivalent to a piece of fruit or about a half a cup of veggies) decreases the risk of heart attack, stroke, and many cancers. No one is telling you to be perfect, but if you know where to aim, you can start to reorganize your kitchen and your trips to the grocery store. It won't take long for your kids to reach for carrots and apples if they are constantly available. Pick pretzels instead of potato chips, and if you have to have chips, then get the baked ones over the regular kind. There are always ways to make improvements. Start small, be realistic, and your family's diet will be better than ever

Get physical — and get your family to go with you. Go for walks. Find a local gym that fits your budget. A lot of centers now offer on-site babysitting and even exercise classes for kids. Look for a health club that's close to home or work, and check the hours to make sure they fit into your schedule. After you join, get your family in the habit of working out at least three or four times a week. If you make it a group activity, you'll be more likely to use your membership. Do whatever you can to build physical activity into your family life, from taking walks after dinner to limiting TV watching, computer time, and video games on weekends.

Don't let the myth that only old people get heart disease and stroke prevent you from taking care of yourself. Even if you know you may be at risk for cardiovascular disease, there is a silver lining. Knowledge gives you a road map, and you can start early to turn things around. While the cheeseburgers of your youth might have helped you get into trouble in the first place, the way you live from now on may help you make amends. The human body is extraordinarily forgiving and constantly tries to repair itself.

NEWS YOU CAN USE

Walking may be the perfect exercise. It's good for your bones, muscles, and flexibility, and it can boost cardiovascular health. It can also keep your knee cartilage healthy and protect against osteoarthritis, according to a study from *Arthritis Care & Research*.

The race to good health is to the moderate. You don't have to give up everything you love to eat, or exercise like you're training for the Olympics. It's the extremes that get us into trouble — either eating everything in sight or dieting or exercising ourselves into walking X-rays. Most of life is played between the forty-yard lines, anyway, and how we eat and how we exercise are no exception. So moderate what you do and stick to a schedule of regular medical checkups. No matter what your circumstances or your age, this is an area very much within your control and it's never too late to get better at being healthy.

Just as there is a silver lining in the prevention and treatment of heart disease, so is there in another disease: cancer. That's where we're headed next.

MYTH #5 . . .

WE'RE LOSING THE WAR ON CANCER

Cancer may be the medical arena most rife with myths, one of the most pervasive being that we're losing the war on cancer. The very phrase *war on cancer* is a misnomer. Cancer is not one disease, but hundreds, with just as many causes and complexities, and each malignancy has its own battle. There are some with real cures, and others that are agonizingly frustrating to detect and treat. On the bright side, we know more about preventing cancer than we ever did before. And increasingly, the treatment of cancer has shifted from not just trying to cure it but also to controlling it as we would any chronic disease, like diabetes, heart disease, even HIV.

Even if a cancer has metastasized and just won't go away, there are so many new drugs and treatments that may slow its growth long enough so that you'll have extra years of relatively good health. You can spend this time being with your family, seeing the

Grand Canyon, continuing to work, devoting yourself to what's important to you — essentially, living life on your own terms. Someone might live for years with a cancer, and should it recur, oncologists can drive it back into remission with another treatment.

I do not want to give you the impression that new drugs and new therapies, or the treatment of cancer as a treatable, controllable disease, means living with cancer is easy — or even doable for some people. How someone lives life with cancer is different from how life is lived with any other disease. Cancer knocks a person off course, and even if you're a five-, ten-, or twenty-year survivor, you still feel as though the sword of Damocles is forever suspended over your head.

I can share with you something that I have observed from my own experience as a surgical oncologist: at a time when you may be fighting for your life, the act of planning for your future and getting on with your life can be a powerful and optimistic experience. I first learned this in 1999, with a patient of mine, Lindsay Beck, who wanted to not only live but also to give life.

Lindsay was just twenty-two years old when she learned that a worsening sore on her tongue was tongue cancer, which was rare for a young person who did not smoke.

Single, she lived in San Francisco and was just starting out in a professional sales career. In her off time, Lindsay was a marathon runner and loved to jog the steep rolling hills of the city.

When the sore did not go away, her doctor suggested that Lindsay see a specialist, Dr. Dan Hartman, who happened to be my partner, and so she made an appointment. Upon examination, Dan didn't like the look of the sore, and so he biopsied the lesion, and the biopsy confirmed that it was cancer.

Lindsay was stunned by the diagnosis. "Who gets cancer in their tongue?" she remembers telling him. "I had never heard of such a thing. I was terrified."

"If you don't mind, I'd like to bring my partner in," Dan recommended. That was when Lindsay officially became my patient.

The cancer that Lindsay suffered from usually occurs in older people who smoke pipes, cigars, and cigarettes or who use smokeless tobacco. Heavy drinking also appears to contribute to the genesis of this malignancy, and men over age sixty develop the disease more often than women. Lindsay's case, of course, was different, since she had none of these risk factors, and it remains a mystery as to why she developed tongue cancer. Fortunately, there were no signs of it

TRUTH

Everyone has a different style of coping with cancer — and that's okay.

There's often pressure placed on cancer patients to adopt a particular attitude in order to improve chances of survival. The idea that your attitude could have an effect on whether you survive cancer picked up steam in the 1980s when some research suggested that survival was longer if you had a "fighting spirit." Other studies said survival may be shortened by an attitude of "helplessness or hopelessness." An actual link between coping styles and cancer, however, has been difficult to prove. To believe that you must adopt a certain attitude to conquer cancer or any other disease can be counterproductive. Suppose you're encouraged to adopt a fighting spirit or think positively, but cancer returns. Does that mean you didn't fight hard enough or do enough positive thinking? You're led to feeling guilty for not having the right attitude, and patient guilt is something I absolutely hate. It's okay to feel, and express, emotions related to cancer — anger, sadness, fear, shock, worry. Don't bottle them up. And regardless of whether or not attitude affects survival, a positive mental outlook can help you improve your quality of life and make constructive decisions about your care.

spreading to the lymph nodes in the neck or to the rest of the body, which is a common occurrence with this type of cancer.

Lindsay, a lean, petite woman with medium ash brown hair, met with me in my office and sat very still. I studied her face, expressionless yet intent, her eyes initially locked in contact with mine. I tried to speak reassuringly, explaining that she would have to treat her cancer. One way was to have surgery and, if necessary, follow it up with radiation and chemotherapy. I told her, too, that she'd have to be involved in her treatment decisions. But as is the case with most patients with a new diagnosis of cancer, her eyes glazed over, and I knew she hadn't digested any of my words. Just hearing the word *cancer* caused her to freeze. There was a lot to absorb, beginning with a diagnosis that didn't make sense.

Finally, I said, "This is a kick in the pants,

but we will get through it together. It is okay to cry."

And she did.

The release of tears brought her attention around. I gave her my cell, office, and home phone numbers, encouraging her to write down any questions she had and call me so that I could answer them.

I explained that she would need surgery — surgery that involved removing over half of her tongue, followed by reconstruction. Lindsay scowled in protest. "I want to be able to talk, eat, even kiss. How can I ever have a normal life with most of my tongue gone?"

I understood her dismay. She was a young woman. Most people who have this surgery are much older and have different quality-of-life concerns. I explained to Lindsay that I had recently treated a prosecuting attorney with the same form of cancer — a woman who thrived on litigating in the courtroom and who demanded that she be able to retain her speech above all else. I gave Lindsay this patient's name and number, and they agreed to meet. Connecting with someone else who had been through the same ordeal helped, and Lindsay took steps toward getting well.

We removed the tumor and part of the

TRUTH

Earwax may predict breast cancer risk.

Ear wax is a buildup of oil and dead skin cells that act like the oil in your car. It lubricates the gentle lining of the ear, keeps your ear moist, and protects it against infection. And contrary to what you might have heard, earwax is not dirty. Talk to anyone who doesn't make enough of it, and they'll tell you how miserable it feels. You should also know that if your earwax has been there since the Nixon administration, it can plug up your ear canals, and it has to be removed, either with an over-the-counter kit or by your doctor. There are two genetically determined types of earwax: dry (which is dry and flaky) and wet (honey brown to dark brown and moist). Most blacks and Caucasians have the wet type while most Asians and Native Americans have the dry type. One of the genetic traits associated with breast cancer is wet earwax. The breasts and the glands that produce earwax are both apocrine glands. According to the Na-

tongue and then put a skin graft in her mouth so that her remaining tongue could move. Radiation followed the surgery. For six weeks, Lindsay received radiation to an area on her body between her nose and her clavicle.

Lindsay did remarkably well with the treatment, and there was no sign of the disease afterward. It seemed that she was cured. She returned to her life but with a new set of priorities. "I no longer wanted to go out partying, or hang out in smoky bars with my twenty-three-year-old friends. I questioned why all of our conversations centered around shoes. There was more to life than that, and I had emerged from my experience with greater wisdom and clarity."

Socially, though, her life became isolating. She was introduced to people, including young eligible men, as "Lindsay, the one who had cancer." "I felt like a Martian with three heads," she complained.

People were defining her by her cancer, though not in a positive way, and so she made the decision to move from San Francisco to New York City, where she could be anonymous and live without the scarlet letter of "cancer survivor" and reclaim her life.

Lindsay remained cancer-free for some eighteen months, after which the cancer returned. She had found a lump in her neck. A needle biopsy of the lump revealed that the cancer had spread to the lymph nodes in her neck. She returned to San Francisco for treatment.

I proceeded to perform a neck dissection. There were no surprises. There was a tumor in her neck, which was the suspicious lump she had felt herself. There was no cancer in her tongue.

In addition to this surgery, I knew that this time around she would require chemotherapy to cut down the chances that this defiant tumor would spread.

Lindsay balked. "I was twenty-four, single, and dating. Not only was my life at stake, but the treatment that could save me might also rob me of my fertility. It was a time in my life when I wanted to fall in love with someone, get married, and have a family. What kind of man would want to marry a two-time cancer survivor — and one who couldn't have babies at that? It was too much to take. I wanted to be left alone."

Lindsay and I were on very different wavelengths. When she said, "I want to get pregnant someday," I just wanted her to get well and live. Her fertility was not my priority. In fact, I wasn't even listening.

Her plan was to become a mom, and I was just getting in her way. To her, cancer was just a speed bump. As she put it, "To me, cancer was temporary. Infertility was permanent, and so that's where I wanted to concentrate my energy."

Lindsay was eventually swayed, however. She underwent chemotherapy and a boost of radiation but not before embarking on a quest to preserve her fertility. "I felt if men could bank their sperm, women should be able to freeze their eggs, and why wasn't anyone talking to me about this?"

At the time, back in 2000, information

TRUTH

Vitamin D is a health builder.

We've known for a long time that vitamin D is good for bones (calcium can't be deposited into bones unless this vitamin is there to help), but a growing body of evidence indicates that it can reduce the risk of premenopausal breast cancer, colon cancer, prostate cancer, and several medical conditions, including osteoporosis, gum disease, diabetes, arthritis, and multiple sclerosis. Vitamin D is normally obtained in adequate amounts through a healthy diet. Some of the richest sources include wild salmon (3 ounces = 420 IU, or international units), Atlantic mackerel (3 ounces = 320 IU), sardines (1 can = 250 IU), shrimp (3 ounces = 150 IU), and shiitake mushrooms (4 pieces = 260 IU). Other good sources are vitamin D–fortified dairy products and cereals.

You also get vitamin D through the skin with ten to twenty minutes of daily sun exposure. But if you slather on a lot of sunscreen (always a good idea) or live in a

Truth, *continued*

rainier, cloudier clime, you're thought to be at a higher risk for a deficiency than those on whom the sun always shines. Should food and sun sources be in short supply, it's a good idea to consider supplements. Take a multivitamin that provides at least the recommended daily value, 400 IU. For women taking extra calcium, buy a brand that also provides vitamin D. The most active — and best — form of vitamin D is D3 (cholcalciferol). Men should not take supplemental calcium, since some research suggests that excessive calcium may increase the risk for prostate concerns.

about cancer and infertility was limited. Yet Lindsay attacked the search for a solution with determination. "I did all the things that most patients do, like scour the Internet, talk to friends and family, ask physicians, and I was really coming up empty-handed." She even went so far as to repeatedly call medical centers, trying to get someone on the line who could give her useful information, and eventually her persistence paid off.

"I finally got someone who knew that

Stanford had an excellent program for cancer patients," Lindsay recalled. "I literally went in the next day for a consultation with a reproductive endocrinologist, and two weeks later my eggs were frozen. At that time, to have people doing whatever they could to make this happen for me, it really made me feel like they thought I would survive. They were actively helping me plan for my future. It was just such a tangible piece of hope."

As Lindsay talked to other young cancer survivors around the country, she'd hear the same story time and time again: none of them had been told by their oncologists that cancer treatment could put them at risk of infertility. "No one knew anything. The cancer world didn't know about fertility and the fertility world didn't know about cancer."

Six months later, with a new lease on life, and a feeling that she had information to share, Lindsay launched a foundation called Fertile Hope, which focused on educating cancer patients about the risks to their fertility and what they could do about it. "I knew there were risks and I knew there were options, and I wanted to get that information out there," she said.

Lindsay did something the medical profession had not: she linked scientists to scien-

TRUTH

You have a better chance of finding skin cancer than your doctor does.

In fact, the chance is twice as probable. That's what researchers at Johns Hopkins University discovered after studying 102 people recently diagnosed with skin cancer. But while doctors were responsible for finding fewer tumors, they found them at an earlier, more treatable stage — because doctors are more meticulous in their screening. These tumors were often lesions on parts of the body that are hard to see yourself, primarily the back, buttocks, and genitalia. They were also much thinner than the ones discovered by patients. This underscores the need for regular all-over skin checks by your doctor, who may spot something that you missed.

When you think about the results of this study, they make sense. Who knows your body better than you? Yet many people shy away from really getting to know what their bodies look like, especially in the most intimate places. And that can spell trouble. Skin cancers, even deadly melanomas, can pop up in places that haven't been exposed to the sun, which is particularly true if you are of a darker-complected skin, as the majority of melanomas discovered within these groups are found in areas that never see the sun.

So get to know your entire body and examine it for suspicious-looking skin growths, including your back, your scalp, the soles of your feet, between your toes. And take a mirror and check all the sensitive areas between your legs. If there are any changes in the size, color, shape, or texture of a mole, or if you develop a new one after age twenty-one, see your doctor.

tists, introducing oncologists to fertility experts.

Since then, Lindsay has carved out quite a glorious life for herself. She met and married Jordan Beck. Two years afterward, she learned she was pregnant after an in vitro fertilization procedure that used a fresh egg from her body; ironically, her frozen eggs had not been needed. She gave birth at the age of twenty-nine to seven-pound, nine-ounce Paisley Jane Beck. As I write this,

TRUTH

You may have encountered articles in the press and on the Internet warning that underarm antiperspirants or deodorants cause breast cancer. The reports suggest that these products contain toxins, which can be absorbed through the skin or enter the body through nicks caused by shaving. To date, however, neither the National Cancer Institute nor the U.S. Food and Drug Administration (which regulates food, cosmetics, medicines, and medical devices) have found any conclusive evidence linking the use of underarm antiperspirants or deodorants and the subsequent development of breast cancer.

Lindsay is pregnant with her second child — and she got pregnant naturally, without any fertility treatments.

Lindsay taught me the importance of getting on with one's life, no matter what the diagnosis. Having something to look forward to doesn't necessarily mean you're going to be cured, but it is important to be able to look past the disease and have something meaningful to focus on. This attitude lets us look to the future, even when the moment we are living is hard, painful, and scary. It rallies our strengths and our natural defenses at those times when we feel most besieged.

ANATOMY OF A MYTH

For background, cancer develops when cells multiply wildly out of order. It is caused by multiple mutations in the genes that control cell division — the process by which a cell duplicates itself by splitting in two. The mutant cell will begin to replicate rapidly, turning into a tumor that might eventually invade surrounding tissue and spread, or "metastasize," to organs where it doesn't belong. There are multiple reasons for cells to become so out of control: age, toxins, genetics, and viruses, among other suspects. Cancer cells are devious, too. By necessity, each generation accumulates more genetic mutations in order to survive — which is why cancer cells often become resistant to the drugs doctors prescribe to kill them. And tumors are able to stimulate their own growth by creating their own nourishing blood supply — a process called angiogenesis.

So you can see why cancer remains such a formidable foe. The fight against it has been on the national agenda since 1971, when President Richard Nixon officially declared war on this dreaded disease. Since then, medicine has made great strides, and consequently, your risk of being diagnosed with cancer and the risk of dying of cancer have decreased significantly. Fewer than half the people diagnosed with cancer today will die of the disease. Some are completely cured, and many more people survive for years with a good quality of life.

So I think there is no question that the war on cancer is being fought and won on multiple fronts — but it is not one "war." Instead, we are battling — and winning — many skirmishes on many battlefronts: in breast cancer, colon cancer, testicular cancer, leukemia, malignant melanoma, and so on. The reason for all the optimism is the life-saving knowledge we've gained in three critical areas: prevention, detection, and treatment.

PREVENTING CANCER

How we live affects our risk for many cancers: lung, colon, skin, breast, prostate, esophagus, stomach, and maybe some other cancers. We smoke and we stay out in the sun too long. We eat too much saturated fat and no-nutrient junk food and too little fiber, and for the most part we are inactive. We also live in a toxic soup of pollution, thanks to our industrialized society. It wasn't always this way; this combustible environmental mix developed over the past few decades, and now these things are part of our daily lives. And now also we are paying the price.

Each year, according to the American Cancer Society, 550,000 Americans die of cancer. One-third of these deaths can be linked to poor diet, lack of physical activity, and being overweight. Smoking, for instance, takes a toll on every organ in your body, from your skin to your bladder, and is linked to at least ten different cancers. How you treated your skin as a teenager can determine if you'll get skin cancer as an adult. Most of the more than one million cases of nonmelanoma skin cancer diagnosed yearly in the United States are related to sun exposure. The number of sunburns you have had over your lifetime dramatically increases your risk for malignant melanoma, the most dangerous skin cancer. The rates for this cancer are increasing in epidemic proportions; it accounts for roughly eleven thousand deaths each year.

TRUTH

Eating sugar does not make cancer spread faster.

All cells, including cancer cells, depend on blood sugar (glucose) for energy. But eating sugar will not speed the growth of cancer cells. Nor will depriving cancer cells of sugar slow their growth. The reason people think sugar makes cancer cells grow faster stems possibly from a misunderstanding of positron emission tomography (PET) scans. Among other uses, doctors use PET scans to assess the spread of tumors. The test involves injecting a small amount of radioactive tracer — typically a form of glucose — into your body. The tracer is absorbed by all tissues of the body. But tissues that are using more energy — like tumors — absorb greater amounts. For this reason, some people have concluded that cancer cells grow faster on sugar. This isn't true.

So if we're increasing our risk of cancer with our own bad habits, changing those habits can be an important first step in cancer prevention. There are preventable risk factors linked to cancer; correcting those things is within our control. We can lower our risk of cancer and stretch out our healthy, productive years by making a few changes in our lifestyle. To me, this takes a lot of the "scare" out of life. What follows are steps you can take to help prevent cancer.

Quit now. There may be no tougher addiction than tobacco. Many health experts now consider nicotine more addictive than heroin. Yet we all know people who have quit, and we know that each person tells a different story as to why he or she quit. There is no easy way to quit, but there have never before been so many options for help. There are many new techniques and tactics available, and some of these include prescription nicotine replacement products such as the nicotine nasal spray Nicotrol inhaler and nonnicotine tablets such as Zyban and the recently approved Chantix. Chantix also partially blocks nicotine from being absorbed by the receptors so smoking is less satisfying. With all these new aids out there to help you quit smoking, it should be easier than ever to kick the habit. But as any ex-smoker can tell you, it is tough. It doesn't matter how you do it: hypnosis, chewing on

TRUTH

Cut back on bacon to cut your risk of stomach cancer.

Bacon, a staple of the American breakfast and low-carb diets, can play a role in stomach cancer. So can sausage or corned beef hash. Research shows that eating just over an ounce of these smoked and processed goodies each day can increase the risk of stomach cancer from 15 percent to 38 percent — perhaps owing to their high salt content, which can irritate the stomach lining, or the nitrate and nitrite additives, which are known carcinogens. Keep your eye on your intake of smoked foods, and limit them as needed.

cinnamon sticks, whatever works for you. Just do it. Be mentally ready, because quitting takes a change of attitude and a lot of inner strength.

Set a date for quitting and try to get a friend or a relative to quit along with you. On the assigned day, stop — no matter what. Be sure to reward yourself each day that you don't smoke: pay yourself. You'll be stunned when you see how much money you're saving. Take the money you save from not buying cigarettes and put it in a jar. Then use that money to treat yourself to a movie, a favorite meal, maybe even a well-deserved vacation.

Overhaul your diet. This could be as simple as cutting back on processed meats like hot dogs and bologna, as well as red meat. Too

TRUTH

A testicular self-exam (TSE) can save a man's life.

One of the most important things a man can do is to examine his testicles monthly for lumps and bumps, much the same way women have been encouraged to perform self-exams for breast cancer. This simple self-exam is the best way to find cancer of the testicles, and many times it is found by a man's partner during sex. This is a cancer that affects men between the ages of fifteen and forty. Testicular cancer is not a common cancer, accounting for only 1 percent of cancers, but it is one of the most curable. As curable as it is, however, over the past fifty years the number of cases has doubled. And research suggests that it's not being caught as early as it could be — another reason for doing TSEs.

To perform this simple procedure, put your index fingers and middle fingers under the testicle and place both thumbs on top. Slowly roll the testicle between your thumbs and fingers. See your doctor if any kind of lump, pain, or discomfort exists.

much red meat may increase your risk of colon and prostate cancers. Load up on vegetables; they may protect you against these and other cancers. Aim for a variety of colored vegetables such as broccoli and peppers. I remember when President George Herbert Walker Bush declared that he didn't like broccoli. I had to smile because he was so insistent, even when broccoli growers around the country cried foul. Broccoli is one of the most perfect vegetables we have. Certain natural chemicals in broccoli and other plant foods boost levels of proteins that repair damaged DNA, and in doing so reduce cancer risk. Fruits and vegetables also fill you up. You can eat as much as you want of them without worrying about the calories.

Trim down. Obesity is linked to many cancers. Excess weight causes the body to produce and circulate more of the hormones estrogen and insulin, which can stimulate cancer growth. Losing weight is easier said than done. If you want to do it successfully, you've got to make friends with food, shun fad diets, eat in moderation, and exercise to keep everything in balance.

Move it. Exercise has its own set of anticancer virtues. If you are looking to prevent cancer, exercise should definitely be a part of

NEWS YOU CAN USE

If you're a guy who loves to chow down on broccoli and cauliflower, you may be less likely to develop aggressive prostate cancer than men who skimp on those vegetables, according to a report published in the *Journal of the National Cancer Institute.*

TRUTH

Stress is a fact of life and it may interfere with the quality of your life, but there is no evidence that everyday stress causes cancer. How do I know? One prestigious medical journal, *The Lancet,* published a review of some seventy studies that collectively looked at stressful life events, particularly loss events, distress level, psychological problems, coping styles, and personality factors. The researchers who analyzed these studies concluded that "there is no psychological factor for which an influence on cancer development has been convincingly shown." I have talked to thousands of patients over the years who have wondered if their stress caused them to get cancer. That thought process is the first step in the "blame game," in which we blame ourselves for something that is usually out of our control. This is a highly detrimental guilt trip that will only make you feel worse psychologically and may distract you from the task at hand — which is to get treated and cured.

your lifestyle. It reduces overweight and obesity, which are linked to an increased risk of cancers of the colon and rectum, breast in postmenopausal women, endometrium, esophagus, and kidney. Evidence is highly suggestive that being overweight also bumps up your risk of cancers of the pancreas, gallbladder, thyroid, ovary, and cervix, as well as multiple myeloma, Hodgkin's lymphoma, and prostate cancer — so being more physi-

TRUTH

Headaches are rarely a sign of a brain tumor.

I wish I had a dollar for every patient I've seen who suspects a headache might be a symptom of a brain tumor. Only very rarely will a headache turn out to indicate a brain tumor. Patients are astounded but mostly relieved when I assure them there is no tumor. If you have recurrent headaches, or a headache that comes on suddenly and feels like something you've never felt before, don't worry, but do see your doctor sooner rather than later so an expert can take a look at what's going on there.

cally active may help lower your risk for many of these. Strenuous exercise, in particular, might be even better. In a study conducted at UCLA, women who exercised aerobically five days a week, an hour each session, had a 20 percent lower risk of invasive breast cancer and a 31 percent lower risk of noninvasive breast cancer, compared with women who exercised less. That said, most of us struggle with finding that much time to exercise every day. So start with simple things such as taking the stairs instead of the elevator or escalator, walking with a friend, gardening, or doing housework. It doesn't really matter how you exercise, but it does matter that you incorporate movement into your everyday life.

Exercise can also be a way to minimize your risk of colon cancer. Exercise accelerates the movement of food through your system, shortening the length of time your digestive tract is exposed to carcinogens. For breast and prostate cancers, it may help by reducing circulating levels of hormones that are associated with tumor growth. If you are undergoing treatment for cancer, or have finished treatment, some level of physical activity can help you overcome fatigue, as well as ease stress and depression. So when it comes to exercise, just do it.

Cover up. Every time you step outside or drive in your car, you are exposed to the sun's rays — even on cloudy or overcast days. Being in the sun feels great, but a little goes a long way. UVB and UVA rays can damage your skin over time and lead to wrinkles and skin cancer. Right now, the Australians are in the midst of a skin cancer epidemic and have developed the "Slip, Slap, Slop" public health campaign. Translation: slip into a long-sleeved shirt, slap on a hat, and slop on some sunscreen. As for sunscreen, make sure you apply it every day, even in the winter. Use a sunscreen with an SPF of at least 30 that clearly states it protects against both UVB and UVA rays, and apply it liberally and evenly over your whole body.

The attitude to take toward cancer prevention is that it's never too late to get better at taking care of yourself. We can't avoid every pitfall in life, but there are enough things we can control, including some risk factors for cancer.

DETECTING CANCER

Early detection is key in dealing with all cancers. As you've read, I'm a big proponent for screening tests and learning all you can about early detection. Even though there are still raging debates about whether early detection reduces death rates or cuts the costs of treating cancer, I err on the side that finding a tumor early is better than detecting it late. When it comes to early detection, no one is more important to the process than you. I can't say it enough, or in too many different ways: don't skip your screening tests — and be sure you know what is recommended for you, based on your sex, personal risk factors, family history, and age. Every day you are alive, some scientist somewhere is a day closer to finding a cure.

What follows is a look at some of the most up-to-date information on cancer screening.

Breast cancer. The standard screening test remains the mammogram, and most doctors will suggest that a woman get one by her fortieth birthday, or sooner if there is a strong family history. If your doctor says you have dense breasts, he or she might suggest a digital mammography. It produces images of the breast that can be enhanced to help doctors better find abnormalities.

Ovarian cancer. As it stands today, there are no great screening tests for ovarian cancer, and this is frustrating. The best defense is an annual pelvic exam in which your gynecologist can feel your ovaries. And there are symptoms to watch for, as I mentioned in chapter 1 (see page 85). A vaginal ultrasound, which can be performed in some doctors' offices, can be a good way of looking at the ovaries. You may have heard of CA-125 for the detection of ovarian cancer. It is not a reliable screening test, however. It recognizes patterns of CA-125 (cancer antigen–125) in the blood, a protein found in elevated levels in most ovarian cancer cells. The test is sensitive but not very specific, and the antigen can be elevated in benign conditions such as pregnancy, endometriosis, pelvic inflammatory disease, and even other cancers. In terms of early detection, CA-125 is elevated in only approximately half the cases of ovarian cancer.

Cervical cancer. Seven strains of the human papillomavirus (HPV) are known to cause cancer of the cervix. In addition to a regular Pap test, your doctor can check for the presence of HPV. HPV and Pap tests are the most accurate way to detect this form of cancer early, and eradicate it before it advances from the cervix. Most doctors advise getting the HPV test every three years, and a yearly Pap test is the norm, in conjunction with a

TRUTH

Millions of Americans — including me — take statin drugs to lower their cholesterol. Now it turns out that taking medicines like Lipitor, Lescol, Pravachol, and Zocor may halve your risk of developing colon and advanced prostate cancers while reducing the risk of pancreatic and esophageal cancers more than 50 percent, according to new research. Doctors also think the cholesterol-lowering and inflammation-reducing benefits of the drugs may help slow the progress of Alzheimer's disease, too.

pelvic exam. Almost every woman with cervical cancer who is diagnosed and treated early can have a good outcome. This is a cancer that can be prevented by getting the HPV vaccine during adolescence, even though the vaccine protects against only four of the seven strains. Being in a monogamous relationship and using condoms if you're not are also protective measures.

Lung cancer. If you are over age fifty and have smoked at least half a pack of cigarettes a day for twenty years or more, it may be prudent to consider a spiral CT, or spiral computed tomography. By rotating around the patient, this lung scan provides three-dimensional images that allow doctors to find many more tiny lung nodules than would be apparent on the standard chest X-ray. It is a sensitive test and can find lung cancer earlier than a standard chest X-ray. It remains to be seen if finding lung cancers early equates to better cure rates. We just don't know yet. Talk to your doctor about whether this test is appropriate for you, and if you're given a thumbs-up, find a testing facility that has experience in lung scanning.

Diagnostic tests continue to evolve. On the near horizon are genetic tests that will be marketed to the public. If you want to, you will be able to get a genetic road map for you, your spouse, and your children, to see who is possibly at risk for cancer. Admittedly, not everyone will want to know, but many will. I have friends who say, "Absolutely not; I do not want to know," and others who say, "Yes, it would be fascinating to find out." These tests may be controversial, and for many may cause consternation,

TRUTH

Cell phones do not cause cancer.

Cell phones operate with radio frequencies, a form of electromagnetic energy. For years scientists have been investigating whether cell phones and electromagnetic fields can cause brain tumors. I admit that the idea of a connection sounds plausible: electromagnetic waves being delivered to a concentrated part of the brain might cause problems. But studies of people who live under high-voltage power lines or near electric substations have so far failed to find a definitive link. Although some people believe that holding a cell phone to your ear for prolonged periods causes brain cancer, there are no studies proving this, either. This is the best we know right now — but it's not the last word. You can be sure of that.

but the technology is here, and soon the tests will be a part of everyday medicine.

Understanding risk factors for cancer and early detection are two of the best weapons we have. Don't be afraid to call your doctor about any suspicious lump or bump or other symptom. Being aware is the first step toward early diagnosis, and early diagnosis is the first step toward successful treatment.

TREATING CANCER

The field of oncology has changed dramatically since I was a young doctor. Cancers such as Hodgkin's lymphoma and acute lymphocytic leukemia in children have largely been defeated and for the most part are now considered curable. Since the 1970s, researchers have amassed a wealth of information about the innermost secrets of malignant cells and how they evolve — which means better methods of targeting treatment are being developed.

The standard treatment for most cancers has been what we unceremoniously call "slash and burn and poison." We surgically excise (slash) all the tumor that we can see and make educated guesses about how much surrounding tissue to remove with the tumor. This is admittedly imprecise and relies on a surgeon's trained eye to tell normal tissue from abnormal tissue combined with a certain surgical insight. Surgery may be followed by radiation (the burn part) and chemotherapy (the poison part). The goal is to kill any errant cancer cells that may have escaped the surgeon's scalpel. These have been the standard treatments now for a couple of decades and remain the basis for most treatment today. I have no doubt that in the future we will look back at surgery with a morbid curiosity and, increasingly, will learn to target cancers in less-invasive ways.

Occasionally, doctors may suggest other ways to treat tumors, including cryotherapy, in which a tumor is frozen, or radio frequency ablation, which destroys tumors with radio waves. Both procedures are less invasive and can have fewer complications.

The biology of targeting tumors is an area that holds extraordinary promise. Today, the new insights into the biological basis of cancer have ignited an explosion into the discovery of new, smarter drugs to fight cancer. For example, we have several drugs in the breast cancer arsenal that you may have heard about. Among them is Herceptin, which interferes with a growth factor by blocking what is called an HER-2 receptor. The HER-2 receptor is found on the surface of many cells but is produced in excessive amounts in some breast cancers.

We know that the biology of various cancers differs from cancer to cancer, which is why interfering with specific tumors at the

TRUTH

Depending on where you live, tap water may be even better for you than the bottled stuff is. While labels prattle on about bottled water coming from mountain spring sources or wells on the slopes of volcanoes, between 25 and 40 percent of bottled water began life less exotically, as tap water. (Bottling companies buy the water and filter it, sometimes pulling minerals and fluoride out in the process.) In most cases tap water adheres to stricter purity standards than does bottled water. Furthermore, studies have found contaminants in bottled water, such as arsenic and carcinogenic compounds in at least some samples at levels exceeding state or industry standards. So enjoy your bottled water when there aren't other options. Relax when the waiter asks you if you want bottled or tap water, knowing that tap water is just fine . . . if not better.

cellular level is another emerging field of treatment. Treatments that accomplish this include targeting growth factors, choking off a tumor's blood supply, and developing anti-cancer vaccines. Gleevec, for example, is a pill that works by targeting and turning off specific proteins in cancer cells that cause these cells to grow and multiply. It has reversed the downhill course of two rare cancers — myelogenous leukemia and a rare form of stomach cancer — for which previously there had been no effective treatments. It is now being tested in other cancers. New drugs like Tarceva and Iressa also block tumor growth by interfering with proteins in cancer cells.

Avastin is the first in a new class of drugs called angiogenesis inhibitors that attack tumors by putting a stop to their ability to create blood vessels, thus starving cancer cells of oxygen and nutrients. And there is a vaccine for melanoma that is injected in an effort to stimulate the immune system to destroy the cancer cells.

Advances like these are being made every day — advances that have taught doctors how to keep the disease at bay for months and sometimes drive it into remission for years. The term *remission* was first used in leukemia and is now applied more loosely in other cancers to denote the shrinkage of a tumor. A more accurate term we doctors use is *no evidence of disease,* or NED, which means that the cancer can no longer be detected by sensitive imaging tests like CT or PET (positron emission tomography) scans. NED doesn't necessarily indicate a *cure* — a term I use very judiciously. It just means that at that moment in time, there is no disease that can be detected. Another term doctors use is "alive with disease." It means that a patient is alive and functioning but that a tumor is present, and it may or may not be interfering with daily activities.

Many of the new anticancer weapons are designed not necessarily to destroy or eliminate wayward cancer cells but instead keep them contained, often with drugs or cocktails of drugs that patients take for the rest of their lives. This strategy of containment is another recent addition to the arsenal of cancer treatment and reflects a welcome shift in the way doctors and patients view cancer.

Case in point: In 2007 Elizabeth Edwards, wife of presidential candidate John Edwards, revealed that she was not just fighting a recurrence of her breast cancer but also wrestling with malignancies that had encamped elsewhere in her body and were no

TRUTH

Your skin is the largest organ of your body.

And an amazing one at that. The skin functions as an endocrine organ, manufacturing hormones like vitamin D for the rest of the body. The skin is also a vital way station of the immune system, filled with specialized white cells that trigger a full-scale immunologic response. The most important thing you can do for your skin is protect it from the sun. As we age our skin gets thinner and drier, so be sure to drink plenty of water and use a good moisturizer. Moisturizers not only hold moisture in the skin but also plump up lines and wrinkles and give the skin a smoother appearance. And while you don't want to become paranoid, you do want to monitor any moles and skin irregularities and inform your doctor of any changes.

longer curable. She has been treated quite intensively in an attempt to contain its further spread. This approach exemplifies this sea change in how doctors and oncologists now view cancer — that it is not a death sentence, and while we may not cure it, we can treat it very aggressively, and in many cases the patient feels pretty well for long stretches of time. The "big C," to my way of thinking, doesn't mean cancer; it means chronic but controllable.

WHAT ABOUT COMPLEMENTARY CANCER TREATMENTS?

Complementary, or integrative (also called alternative), medicine includes lifestyle changes like diet, exercise, and vitamin therapy — which all of us to some degree should do on a daily basis. It also includes acupuncture, massage, chiropractic medicine, relaxation therapy, herbal medicine, and more. As a doctor, I've seen patients who were helped enormously by such therapies, particularly in conjunction with mainstream medicine, and I've seen patients embrace forms of complementary medicine as if they were cure-alls for cancer and come away hurt and disappointed.

It is human nature to pin our hopes on any new remedy or treatment that comes out, but of course we can't. Most treatments, conventional or complementary, have chinks somewhere. We just have to be judicious and employ common sense. Many complementary therapies do have a place in the treatment of cancer and other diseases. Among them are acupuncture to reduce pain; art therapy to help patients express emotions; massage to ease stress, anxiety, and depression; meditation to relax the body and calm the mind; and music therapy to promote healing. Prayer and spirituality can be a powerful force for health, too. Questions of spirit and soul are very personal, but when asked whether I buy into the notion that faith creates healing energy, I answer "Definitely." Faith and spirituality are intensely personal. We simply need to find for ourselves what spiritual pattern gives our lives the most meaning.

As for supplements, almost every day some new vitamin or supplement promises to be the next miracle cure. But the science is always evolving. There is now evidence that getting sufficient vitamin D, including from sunlight (its natural source), may cut your risk of breast cancer in half, and the American Cancer Society reported in one study that people who took a calcium supplement were 30 percent less likely to develop colon cancer than those who didn't. (For more on the subject of supplements, see chapter 6.)

Should you be diagnosed with a life-

TRUTH

"Light" cigarettes are just as harmful to your health as "regular" brands.

Fewer than 10 percent of smokers are aware that 1 light or ultralight cigarette yields the same amount of tar as one regular cigarette, according to a report published in the *American Journal of Public Health*. Despite decades of the tobacco industry advertising light cigarettes that claim to have lower tar and nicotine content, there is no meaningful difference in smoke exposure or health risks among cigarettes with different tar and nicotine yields. Light cigarettes deliver the same amounts of tar, nicotine, and carbon monoxide to smokers as standard brands. Many people who use low-tar, light, or ultralight cigarettes tend to smoke more cigarettes and inhale smoke harder and deeper into their lungs, increasing the dangers all the more.

threatening illness like cancer, you'll need support. Don't shy away from asking for help from friends and family. Whether you get the support you need from your loved ones, you will also want to consider support groups (as well as seeking help from a social worker, therapist, counselor, or religious mentor). Almost every cancer care center in the United States offers support groups. In a support group you can learn coping skills to reduce anxiety, depression, fatigue, and pain, plus how to better control your life and your treatment. Some research into the value

TRUTH

Eating grilled or pan-fried meats can increase your risk of cancer.

Grilling or pan-frying meat creates chemicals called heterocyclicamines (HCAs), which can be harmful. These chemicals are found in higher quantities when meat is well done or burned. Experts recommend limiting the amount of grilled meat in your diet and avoiding the burned parts altogether. To cut down on HCAs, marinate and precook meats in a microwave before cooking by other methods. Many grilled foods are safe and good for you, including grilled vegetables and fruits.

of support groups for cancer patients has shown that group psychotherapy may extend lives, but more recent studies have shown otherwise. Whether or not there is a survival benefit, this type of therapy is very important to cancer care. Even if support groups don't help someone live longer, they can improve quality of life by alleviating some of the side effects of cancer treatment.

I also believe in psychoneuroimmunology (PNI). This is the study of how thoughts and emotions affect the immune system. I was introduced to PNI long before it was codified into a science, when my own father employed it after he was diagnosed with colon cancer. Using visual imagery, he imagined his immune system as a factory pumping out little PAC-MAN figures that would march through his body, gobbling up cancer cells. I was amazed to see this traditionally trained surgeon, in his sixties at the time, with his life jeopardized by colon cancer, turning to this form of meditation. He was so ahead of the times. He willed the cancer cells to die. Try visualization techniques as my father did, or "guided imagery," often described as "directed daydreaming," a form of visualization led by another person or on a CD or audiotape. They can help you reduce stress or anxiety, manage the chronic pain, and potentially assist in the healing process.

Hold on to hope. It can come from a friend, a relative, your children, or the doctors and nurses at the practice where you're getting your care — anyone with whom you feel safe and comfortable. Watch comedies, since laughter has been known to relieve stress and make you feel uplifted. Employ affirmations or start journaling, both of which have had striking effects in patients with whom I've worked. The sheer power of participating in your own healing can be very strong medicine.

Complementary and integrative medicine, as well as supplements, can cohabitate peacefully with conventional medical care, as long as you know the facts and can distinguish what's credible and what's a crock. Ideally, the treatments you select should work together with the care of your conventional doctor. For your safety, always tell your doctor about any complementary medicine treatments you use.

FOLLOW UP WITH YOUR DOCTOR

Once you have been diagnosed and treated for cancer, you play a very important role in making sure you remain healthy. You must continue to see your doctor. Many people find this difficult to do and put off appointments because of the very natural fears they have regarding recurrence. Put your fears on hold and keep your appointments. I keep a very tight rein on my cancer patients — and I hope your doctor does, too. I see mine once a month for a year, then every three months, then every six months, then once a year. Even if the visit consists of a mere fifteen minutes annually, my patients always have a ticket to the front office. Seeing less of your doctor over time means you are moving in the right direction.

Between advancements in prevention and treatment, the advent of new drugs, and continued efforts at improved diagnostic techniques, the future for cancer patients looks better and better. There is a huge amount of information you'll find, whether from accessing the Internet or talking to experts. Many times, this helps; at others, it clouds the picture. The best thing to do is listen to your doctors and listen to your gut. Having a voice and a partnership with your doctor is the best way to deal with the curveball of a cancer diagnosis.

Supposed cure-alls for diseases like cancer, heart disease, and even aging are coming from many directions, and none are more controversial than those dubbed natural remedies. But what's the real story? Are these curative measures worth considering or not? They might indeed work, but are they safe? Keep turning the page, and I think you'll be surprised by the answers.

MYTH #6 . . .

NATURAL MEANS "SAFE"

I've encountered many patients over the years who have wrestled with accepting established medical advice versus using some "natural" remedy for their health problem. If a product is "natural" and doesn't require a prescription, then it must be safe, good for you, low in side effects, and tied to longevity, right? Not necessarily. Tobacco is natural, for example, but we know it's a slow killer. So is arsenic. Still, people say, "I don't want to take a drug, Dr. Snyderman. Isn't there something natural I can take?"

Earlier in my medical career, I didn't have a good answer for such questions. Most of my patients in Little Rock took what I prescribed for them and stayed the course, not veering off onto nontraditional healing paths. But when I moved to San Francisco, patients were different. They told me they were using this or that — herbs and supplements I had never heard of. I would dissuade my patients from taking them and tell them that they were wasting their money, that the stuff they were putting in their mouths was worthless. But I made one cardinal error. I had no more proof when I told them what not to take than they did when deciding to take it.

One day a lightbulb just went on: I could learn something about this exploding field of supplementation. Or I could stick my head in the sand while my patients megadosed, detoxified, juiced, whatever — without ever divulging their secrets, because there would be no motivation or dialogue to share their true medical histories (which I needed to know in order to treat them properly). I didn't think I was practicing the best medicine I could because I was unwilling to listen. And my patients were treating themselves in spite of me, not with me. I came to realize that I owed my patients more.

With that, I read, spoke with doctors, and took courses in an effort to learn more. I listened to my patients and took off the blinders. I wanted to know what my patients were taking, and I wanted them to know I had an open mind.

Many people feel they have been helped by taking supplements; others feel their time and their money have been wasted. The truth is that there are times when supplements can complement care and other times when they can conflict with the treatments and medications we doctors prescribe. Remember the patient Lindsay I told you about in chapter 5? Cancer patients like Lindsay are easy prey for unjustified hope and promises. They feel desperate and want to do something for themselves, something proactive and empowering. And so, it is understandable that after Lindsay's cancer diagnosis and treatment she would try anything and everything to get a full guarantee against a recurrence of her disease. Her mother had tipped me off that Lindsay was taking a lot of things, from megavitamins to herbal tonics, and she was justifiably concerned. Her mother just wanted to make sure that none of them would hurt her. For her next appointment, I asked Lindsay to bring in her "medicines" so I could take a look. She came in with a grocery bag, filled to the top. She dumped everything out, and it looked like she had bought out an entire health-food store. There were vitamins, energy drinks, dried herbs, capsules, pills, powders, gels, and lotions. Most, even though in doses I found way too high, weren't going to hurt her, but I had no faith that they were going to cure her cancer. Plus, she was taking many of these supplements in megadoses that the body can't even absorb. They were washing through her body, doing no real good and instead producing pretty expensive urine. The other problem — the one that worried me the most — was that Lindsay was taking so many supplements that she had almost forgotten to eat real food or enjoy a meal, which was jeopardizing her health. She was consumed to the point of obsession with these nostrums, and she had forgotten there was a life to live — hers.

I suggested that she toss most of her supplements out with the garbage, keep a few of her favorites, and go out and get a chocolate milkshake. She burst into tears of relief. That afternoon, she drank a huge, frothy milkshake. "It was delicious," she told me.

ANATOMY OF A MYTH

Lindsay fell into the trap that many of us have at one time or another — taking a do-it-yourself approach to medicine. This is an ever-growing phenomenon, and no wonder. The marketing of supplements is alluring and aggressive, with unchallenged claims that suggest healing powers or the latest in scientific "miracle" ingredients for everything from curing arthritis and cancer to guaranteeing weight

TRUTH

Doctors like alternative medicine.

A recent survey of Mayo Clinic doctors found that by and large physicians agree that a number of alternative medicine therapies hold promise for the treatment of symptoms and diseases. And more than 64 percent of medical schools are teaching some form of alternative medicine. Until 1988, when I first moved to San Francisco from Little Rock, Arkansas, I knew very little about "alternative" medicine. In fact, all I really knew was what I had read, and as a classically trained physician, what I read I mistrusted.

But all that began to change when I made a trip to Arizona to shoot a story with Dr. Andrew Weil, a physician and now-noted expert in the field of complementary and alternative medicine. He went to Harvard Medical School and then studied contemporary shamanism in South America, calling shamans the "doctors of bodies, souls, and situations." I watched him in action and observed how he practiced this

Truth, *continued*

"alternative" medicine. I found it wasn't so alternative after all. For patients who had stuffy noses, he prescribed freeze-dried stinging nettles, cautioning that this herb wouldn't work as quickly as some of the over-the-counter antihistamines but wouldn't have the side effects, either. I watched him counsel a patient who had traveled across the country to get a second opinion for a cancer. It would have been easy for a lesser doctor to prescribe an herb or a potion and send this chap on his way. Instead, Andy told him that he needed a surgeon — and fast. For follow-up, Andy invited him back to try some natural therapies to alleviate the side effects of cancer treatment, such as nausea, vomiting, or loss of energy. Andy explained to me that what he does is not alternative at all but rather *integrative,* a word I now prefer and use myself. It means welding conventional medical treatments with alternative treatments that have good studies of safety and effectiveness behind them. Watching his commonsense approach, and studying alternative methods on my own, I became a believer, joining legions of other doctors who believe, too.

loss. Add to this the fact that more and more of us are quite wary about invasive medical techniques, the high costs and side effects of prescription drugs, and the often emotionless care received by overworked, frazzled doctors in this day of managed care medicine, and you can see why so many people are embracing natural healing techniques with greater frequency.

The use of natural remedies is not really a new phenomenon; they have been with us since the beginning of time. Ancient healers washed wounds in beer, made poultices out of lizard dung, and used incantations and amulets to drive out evil spirits. Then came Hippocrates, the famed Greek father of medicine, with his own take on natural medicine, announcing, "If we could give every individual the right amount of nourishment and exercise, not too little and not too much, we would have found the safest way to health." Of course, we all know these things, but it was Hippocrates who knew them first. It was Hippocrates who also said, "First do no harm."

In this day and age, most consumers think natural products are harmless and safe — and I can understand why. Herbs, for example, are natural. An herb is a flower, leaf, or stem; a seed or root; a fruit or the bark, or

TRUTH

Hyperactivity in kids is not related to sugar.

There's no scientific evidence that sugar triggers hyperactivity in children. But it will make them obese. Moreover, many high-sugar foods are loaded with fat, so if your kids are eating a lot of sugar- and fat-laced foods, they'll start putting on pounds, even to the point of being at greater risk for "adult" diseases like type 2 diabetes and heart disease. It's wise to reduce sugar in your family's diet. No matter how good it tastes, it's just not good for us.

any part of a plant that is used for its flavor, medicinal, or odiferous properties. The word *drug* comes from the Middle English *drogge,* "to dry," as dried plants were often used as medicines. You've probably practiced some form of herbal medicine, whether you know it or not. If you've sipped a cup of tea, for example, you've had an herbal remedy.

Consumers take for granted that as with pharmaceutical drugs, some government agency tests all natural products to be sure that they are safe and effective and puts them through an approval process. This is not true. In 1994, in response to forceful lobbying on the part of supplement makers, Congress passed the Dietary Supplement Health and Education Act, which changed the way the industry was regulated. Now vitamins, minerals, herbs, and other "natural" substances you see on the shelves do not need review or approval from the U.S. Food and Drug Administration (FDA) before going on the market. As part of this act, supplement manufacturers were told that they must be able to substantiate the safety of their ingredients. This has not been enforced until recently. The agency phased in the rule requiring supplement makers to test the purity and composition of their products. Large companies are doing this now, but smaller companies have until 2010 to comply.

Still, we'll continue to be hard-pressed to know for sure whether certain supplements are truly safe or effective. Since nutritional supplements contain naturally occurring compounds that cannot be easily patented, there is little incentive for drug companies to do extensive and expensive studies to prove safety and effectiveness. And without studies, many mainstream physicians will not embrace them.

Already we know that some of these remedies can be downright dangerous — even deadly. A manufacturing problem led the U.S. government to ban the popular sleep supplement L-tryptophan, an amino acid, in 1990 after contaminated pills led to a rare muscle disease that sickened thousands and killed more than thirty Americans. In 2004 the FDA banned dietary supplements containing ephedrine alkaloids (ephedra) because they posed a risk of serious adverse events, including heart attack, stroke, and death. The prior year, I remember reading about one of these deaths — the heatstroke death of twenty-three-year-old Baltimore Orioles pitcher Steve Bechler. A medical examiner believed his death was at least partly caused by an ephedra supplement he took — a tragic reminder of why *natural* doesn't necessarily mean "safe."

Also in 2004 the Consumers Union, the independent nonprofit publisher of *Consumer Reports,* warned Americans that they should avoid a "dirty dozen" of supplements that may cause cancer, heart problems, kidney or liver damage, even death. On the list were aristolochic acid (snakeroot), comfrey, androstenedione, chaparral, germander,

TRUTH

Bread is good for you.

Bread is called the staff of life for a reason. It has nourished humans in numerous cultures for centuries. It hasn't been until the past few years that we have demonized bread — and there's a reason. We stripped bread of most of its natural nourishment and complexity when plastic-wrapped white bread was introduced to the U.S. market. That new bread was cheap and didn't go stale quickly, but it was high in simple, low-nutrient carbohydrates and sugar and packed very little nutritional punch.

Personally, I think bread is one of the greatest gifts on earth and should be consumed with great joy. Today you can get fresh breads just about anywhere. When buying bread, look for those with at least 2 grams of fiber per slice. Stick with whole-wheat and whole-grain forms of bread, and don't hesitate to freeze half the loaf if you are worried about keeping it fresh.

kava, bitter orange, over-the-counter organ/glandular extracts (thought to increase the risk of mad cow disease particularly from brain extracts), lobelia, pennyroyal oil, skullcap, and yohimbe.

With some supplements the watchword is caveat emptor: let the buyer beware. In recent years, multiple private labs have tested supplement quality, only to find out that some manufacturers fail to deliver what's promised on their product labels. For example, tests have shown that certain formulations of supplements lacked advertised ingredients, including chondroitin, saw palmetto, and coenzyme Q-10. Each is pricey, and many are supplied by China, a country with a long tradition of herbal remedies but, as we know from recent news reports, a poor record of food and supplement safety. Similar tests have found some supplements tainted with potentially harmful ingredients such as lead, pesticides, and bacteria; a few have even been found to harbor prescription drugs. What you're buying may not contain what it is advertised to contain, and you may get more (or less) than you bargained for.

We want to put our faith in the new remedies and treatments that come out, but of course we can't. Most treatments, supplemental or pharmaceutical, have chinks somewhere. We just have to be judicious and employ common sense. Some supplements are worthwhile, as long as you know the facts and can distinguish what's credible and what's a crock. What I'll do here is describe for you what I like about certain supplements — and what to avoid — in the hopes of demystifying what may prove useful, viable alternatives for you.

HERBAL MEDICINE

Herbs can be as powerful as mainstream medicine. Surprised I say this?

About 25 percent of all prescription drugs are derived from trees, shrubs, or herbs. Taxol — a potent chemotherapeutic drug — is isolated from the bark of the Pacific yew tree. Aspirin comes from willow trees, and digitalis (a heart medicine) from foxglove. Birth control pills originated from the Mexican yam.

Herbs are not as well studied as prescription drugs, despite their age-old uses in traditional medicine from cultures all around the world. But herbs certainly do make the news. Every time you turn around you hear another claim for an herb. A good example is echinacea. This very popular herb got a second look recently when the prestigious medical journal *The Lancet* published a report that said echinacea decreases the odds of getting a cold by 58 percent. Yet other previously published studies on this herb hadn't painted such a rosy picture of its cold-fighting powers. One study, funded a few years ago by the National Institutes of Health, said that it just doesn't work. So as you already know with many things medical: the research into herbs tends to be contradictory, so many herbs remained unproved.

One category of herbal remedies I have often warned against are those promoted for weight loss. Go anywhere and you'll see countless ads appealing to our desire to be thin or thinner. Many of these supplements claim to boost your metabolism (the rate at which you expend calories), tame your appetite, and burn fat. These supplements are put together with a variety of stimulants — mostly herbal — alone or in a blend, such as caffeine (typically in the form of guarana, kola nut, or yerba maté) or ephedrine (as ephedra), which as I noted earlier can cause severe, often fatal side effects. Other ingredients commonly used in herbal weight-loss formulas include: garcinia cambogia, which supposedly suppresses appetite (though research shows no evidence that it works for weight loss in humans); and bitter orange, a

TRUTH

One to 3 cups of joe a day helps retain memory.

If anyone knows the importance of a boost from caffeine, it's me in the morning. Now it turns out that caffeine may help me remember where I put my car keys. In November 2005, Austrian researchers confirmed that caffeinated coffee can *temporarily* sharpen your focus and memory. After giving volunteers the caffeine equivalent of about 2 cups of coffee a day, their brain activity was increased in two locations — the memory-rich frontal lobe and the attention-controlling anterior cingulum.

Caffeine is not for everyone. Avoid caffeine if you suffer from restlessness, anxiety, irritability and/or headaches, or sleep problems; gastrointestinal problems; irritable bowel syndrome or ulcers; elevated blood pressure or abnormal heart rhythms; or premenstrual syndrome or fibrocystic breasts.

TRUTH

Colon cleansing, or colonics, is a procedure that involves having an enema or using a laxative that completely evacuates the intestine. It has been touted as everything from a toxin remover to a cure for cancer. Some spas even offer the treatment. Use of enemas particularly scares me because it may involve unskilled personnel performing a procedure that could be harmful.

Not only does colon cleansing provide no benefit, it can be downright dangerous. There is a real risk of damaging the rectum and even perforating the bowel. Contrary to popular belief, the inside of the colon — the end of the large intestine — isn't dirty and does not need to be cleaned out. Mother Nature does that on her own by making sure that waste passes through and out of your body, taking impurities with it. If you want to flush out impurities from your body, have another glass of water instead.

stimulant that may be dangerous, especially when used by the elderly, the obese, and those with cardiovascular disease.

With products like these, we are being sold a bill of goods — that if you just pop one of these pills, you will lose weight — as if the supplement were a magic bullet. The truth is the only magic bullet to weight loss is what no one wants to hear: changing your daily routine to make exercise and a healthy, low-calorie, nutrient-dense diet a lifelong habit.

Despite their botanical names and woodsy packaging, herbs can be potent medications. People are mixing them with over-the-counter medications, prescription drugs, and other medical treatments, trying to cure themselves, but sometimes oblivious to the fact that they could be making themselves sicker. (See the Common Herb–Drug Interactions chart on pages 288–292 for the ways in which herbs and drugs can interact adversely with one another.)

I always ask my patients who are scheduled for surgery what medicines and supplements they are taking, since a number of popular products can cause serious side effects during surgery. Some examples: Saint-John's-wort, which many people take to relieve depression, anxiety, and insomnia, can intensify the effects of some anesthetics and narcotics. Ginkgo biloba, which is used to improve memory, and feverfew, a headache treatment, can reduce the number of blood platelets, which are necessary for clotting. Ginseng, touted to increase vitality, among other things, has been associated with both high blood pressure and accelerated heart rate during surgery. The safest thing to do is tell your doctor everything you are taking (and tell the anesthesiologist, too) and stop using all herbals two (better yet, three) weeks before surgery; this should be enough time for any medicines to clear from your body. If you can't, at least bring the bottles of any medication, pharmaceutical and herbal, to

NEWS YOU CAN USE

Get your vitamin A naturally — from a carrot. One 7-inch carrot contains 600 micrograms of vitamin A, also known as retinol. That's close to our daily requirement for this nutrient: men need 900 micrograms a day; women, 700 micrograms. Excess amounts of vitamin A in pill form can be toxic, potentially causing blurred vision, headaches, vomiting, and problems to the bones, liver, and central nervous system.

the hospital with you. The labels can provide important information to your doctors.

Not all herbs are bad guys. Some are fairly benign and may have therapeutic value. Aloe applied topically is great for soothing the inflammation of a sunburn. Raspberry tea may ease menstrual cramps and diarrhea. Chewing a teaspoon of fennel seeds helps relieve gas after a meal. Cranberry juice may help keep your urinary tract healthy. I recommend a few herbal remedies myself, such as stinging nettles for the alleviation of hay fever symptoms, ginger for motion sickness, and green tea for its antioxidant value. I have used arnica for deep bruises. I eat garlic occasionally too, which is great for my heart and it tastes good. (And believe it or not, garlic does wonders for my marriage. I love it when my husband says, "You look thinner from a distance.")

Today, there is certainly no shortage of herbal products available. Go to any pharmacy or health food store and you'll stand before the "great wall" of herbal remedies. It can be overwhelming, so here's my advice on taking herbs: we don't have all the answers yet, but what we do know is that herbal medicines work in the same manner that pharmaceutical drugs work — they may work, they have their own side effects, and they can

COMMON HERB–DRUG INTERACTIONS

Herb	Common Use	May Interact With	Potential Effects
Arnica	Wound healing, bruise treatment	Blood pressure medicines, blood thinners	Decreases the effects of these drugs
Black cohosh	Treatment for hot flashes, premenstrual discomfort	Estrogen, oral contraceptives	May decrease the body's response to these drugs
Cascara	Laxative	Cardiac glycosides, such as digitalis, and thiazide diurietics	Causes loss of potassium with chronic use; can dangerously increase the effects of cardiac glycosides
Chamomile	Mild sedative; anti-inflammatory	Iron, blood thinners	Blocks iron absorption and may interfere with the action of blood thinners

Ephedra	Treatment for obesity and asthma	Blood pressure drugs, cardiac glycosides	Increases blood pressure; may overstimulate the central nervous system
Evening prim- rose oil	Treatment for high cholesterol, breast tenderness, eczema	Anticonvulsants, anti- Parkinson drugs	May increase the risk of seizures in patients taking medicine to lower seizure threshold
Feverfew	Migraine prevention	Iron, blood thinners	Blocks iron absorption and may interfere with the action of blood thinners
Garlic	Treatment for abnor- mal blood lipids	Blood thinners, oral diabe- tes drugs	May increase the effects of both drugs (not always a positive)
Ginkgo biloba	Treatment for demen- tia and to improve circulation	Blood thinners, anticonvul- sants, tricyclic antidepres- sants	Increases the effects of blood thinners; may increase the risk of seizures

COMMON HERB–DRUG INTERACTIONS

Herb	Common Use	May Interact With	Potential Effects
Ginseng	Stimulant	Blood thinners, cardiac drugs, blood pressure drugs, estrogen replacement drugs, diabetes drugs, antidepressants	May increase or decrease the effects of any of these drugs
Guarana	Stimulant	Blood thinners	Increases the effects of blood thinners
Kava	Treatment for anxiety and sleep disorders	Alcohol, sedatives	Increases the effects of sedatives; can be toxic to the liver
Kelp	Treatment for obesity, thyroid dysfunction	Thyroid hormones	May interfere with thyroid replacement

Red clover	Treatment for menopause symptoms	Blood thinners, oral contraceptives	May increase the risk of bleeding; interferes with oral contraceptives
Saint-John's-wort	Treatment for depression	Antidepressants, iron, piroxicam (an anti-inflammatory) and photosensitizers (drugs that make your skin sensitive to the sun)	May increase blood pressure, interfere with antidepressants, block iron absorption, and increase the risk of sunburn
Saw palmetto	Treatment for benign prostate enlargement	Iron, estrogens	May block iron absorption; may increase the effects of estrogen
Senna	Laxative	Diuretics, cardiac glycosides	Causes loss of potassium with chronic use; increases the effects of cardiac glycosides

COMMON HERB–DRUG INTERACTIONS

Herb	Common Use	May Interact With	Potential Effects
Valerian	Sedative	Sedatives	May increase the effects of prescription sedatives
Yohimbe, yohimbine	Treatment for impotence	Blood pressure medication, antidepressants	May induce hypotension or hypertension, and irregular heartbeat when taken with blood pressure drugs; may interfere with antidepressants

Sources: A. A. Izzo et al., Cardiovascular pharmacotherapy and herbal medicines: The risk of drug interaction, International Journal of Cardiology 98 (2005): 1–14; A. A. Izzo and E. Ernst, Interactions between herbal medicines and prescribed drugs: A systematic review, Drugs 61 (2001): 2163–2175; G. Valli et al., Benefits, adverse effects and drug interactions of herbal therapies with cardiovascular effects, Journal of the American College of Cardiology 39 (2002): 1083–1095; J. F. Villegas et al., Adverse effects of herbal treatment of cardiovascular disease: What the physician must know, Heart Disease 3 (2001): 169–175; and R. A. Vogel et al., ACCF Complementary medicine expert consensus document, Journal of the American College of Cardiology 46 (2005): 184–221.

TRUTH

Sorry, tomato lovers. There is no credible evidence that these foods, which contain a healthy antioxidant called lycopene, prevent lung, colorectal, breast, cervical, or uterine cancer, and there is only very limited evidence that tomatoes can reduce the risk of prostate, ovarian, gastric, and pancreatic cancers. This finding is straight from the mouth of the U.S. Food and Drug Administration, which in 2007 evaluated 145 studies of lycopene, tomato, or tomato product intake and cancer risk to arrive at its conclusion. Does this mean you shouldn't eat these foods? Not at all. When used as part of a diet that includes lots of other brightly colored vegetables, they're beneficial for your health. But do they prevent you from getting cancer? I won't go that far.

interact with other drugs. If you have questions or are considering an herbal supplement, look into whether the herb reacts with anything, especially any medicines you're taking, note any side effects it may have, and don't be afraid to tell your doctor the truth.

NATURAL HORMONE REPLACEMENT

I get a lot of questions from women on the use of natural remedies for menopause — and no wonder. For approximately two-thirds of all women, this natural passage of life is filled with discomforts — hot flashes, night sweats, mental fuzziness, vaginal dryness, loss of libido, weight gain, and more. A deficiency of estrogen in our bodies causes most of the noticeable symptoms of menopause. Estrogen or hormone replacement therapy (HRT) was thus heralded as the standard of care, until one arm of a federally funded study called the Women's Health Initiative was halted early because researchers found that women taking estrogen and progesterone had more heart attacks, strokes, blood clots, and breast cancer. This stunned many doctors who believed that HRT was here to stay. Patients were equally stunned, and many started pinning their hopes on natural means for relief. Sales of prescription FDA-approved hormones plummeted, creating a demand for "bioidentical hormone replacement therapy." Its sales pitch is a hard one to resist, with one endorser calling it "the juice of youth," and a commercial touting it as the "more natural alternative."

Bioidenticals are custom-made chemicals designed in a lab by pharmacists who say they use the same molecular recipe a woman's body uses to create her own hormones. There are about three thousand pharmacies in the United States that fill orders for custom-made hormonal compounds, and they get their ingredients from the same suppliers the drug companies do. Typically, bioidentical hormones contain three estrogens (estrone, estradiol, and estriol), progesterone, and androgens such as testosterone or dehydroepiandrosterone (DHEA) and are usually formulated as a cream rubbed onto the skin, liquids given as drops, or as troches, which are small, circular lozenges.

But are they any safer than traditional HRT?

I do not believe they are. While they are being promoted to consumers as safe alternatives to conventional menopausal hormone therapy, and as health-promoting tonics, no reliable data yet support these claims. A recent study published in the *Medical Journal of Australia* reported on three women who developed endometrial cancer after taking bioidentical HRT to relieve menopausal symptoms. Many of the country's most esteemed medical organizations, such as the American Medical Association, the Endocrine Society, and the North American Menopause Association, have come out with statements of reservation about bioidenticals. The FDA, which can regulate these compounds, is taking a closer look at compounded bioidentical products.

For short-term use (three to five years), these products may be a reasonable treatment for the symptoms of perimenopause (premenopause), the phase before menopause actually takes place, when ovarian hormone production is on the wane and fluctuating, producing a host of symptoms, such as hot flashes, night sweats, and vaginal dryness. It is the prolonged use of hormones well after menopause that concerns me.

At the end of the day, no one can decide if HRT, even bioidentical HRT, is right for you except you and your doctor, based on your health and personal risk factors. The choice is yours to make in consultation with your doctor.

HOMEOPATHY

Founded in the late eighteenth century by Samuel Hahnemann, a German physician, homeopathy is an alternative therapeutic system based on the principle that like cures like or the law of similars. This means that what you have is that which you are given in small doses. This is the same principle behind most vaccines: your being infected with a minute amount of a virus helps your body's immune system defend against the virus.

Another law in homeopathy is the law of the infinitesimal dose, which holds that the more a remedy is diluted, the greater its potency. On homeopathic containers, you'll see such notations as 10X, or 80X or even 30C. Each X signifies that the active substance has undergone a ten-to-one dilution; each C a hundred-to-one dilution.

A third principle is that any illness or condition you suffer from will have unique characteristics common only to you, and remedies are selected on that basis. So if you have

TRUTH

Here's a condition that can respond well to natural treatments: heartburn. Although some sixty million Americans suffer from heartburn — twenty-five million of them every day — most don't understand what's causing their misery. As a result, say researchers from New York's Memorial Sloan-Kettering Cancer Center, people tend simply to pop antacids without taking steps that might eliminate the problem. Not everyone is bothered by the same things, but it's worth trying the following suggestions.

- **Don't go to bed with a full stomach.** Heartburn occurs when acid from your stomach leaks through the muscular valve separating the stomach from the esophagus and makes its way into your chest and throat, where it produces burning and a squeezing sensation. If you eat a large meal late in the evening, you'll be lying flat when your stomach is producing most of the acid necessary for digestion, making it easier for the acid to leak.

- **Watch how much you drink.** Alcohol increases the amount of stomach acid you produce; with a late meal, it's a double whammy.
- **Keep your hands off the chocolate mints.** Those chocolate mints that are so hard to resist after dinner not only increase stomach acid, they also relax the sphincter that keeps the stomach contents where they belong.
- **Sleep on a couple of pillows.** Gravity is your friend: when your head is higher than your stomach, it will help the stomach acids to stay in your stomach and not back up into your throat.

a cold, and your symptoms are watery eyes and a thin, clear nasal discharge, a homeopath might treat you with a remedy prepared from onion extract because these symptoms mimic those produced by onions. Someone else with a cold might have a thick,

TRUTH

Sports drinks may cause irreversible damage to teeth.

Sports drinks, a popular liquid supplement, contain organic acids that attack the hard outer enamel of the tooth's surface and cause damage three to eleven times greater than that caused by soda, according to a report in the journal *General Dentistry*. Once the enamel has been penetrated, the softer dentin beneath is attacked, and tooth decay sets in. You can minimize the decay-producing effects of these drinks by cutting back on or limiting them, or by chugging them rather than sipping.

yellow discharge and be treated with a different homeopathic remedy.

Is there a difference between homeopathy and herbal medicine? Yes. Herbal medicine is just that — medicine made from herbs. Although homeopathy uses herbs, it also uses animal matter and other substances. For example, the homeopathic remedy Oscillococcinum, used to treat flu, is manufactured from wild duck heart and liver, believed to be reservoirs for influenza viruses (which might make you think flu shots aren't such a bad idea after all).

Homeopathy is controversial. In an article published in 1991 in the *British Medical Journal,* in which 107 clinical studies of homeopathic remedies were reviewed, it was reported that 81 of these studies found that homeopathy was beneficial in treating such conditions as headaches, digestive problems, respiratory infections, sprains, and postoperative infections. But in a more recent review study, published in 2005 in *The Lancet,* researchers compared the results of 110 trials of homeopathy with the same number of trials of conventional medicine. The conclusion: benefits credited to homeopathy were, at best, placebo effects.

Some classic homeopathic physicians believe that homeopathy can replace the need for standard childhood vaccinations. Not so. Homeopathy cannot protect children from communicable childhood diseases. Children need to be immunized against these diseases. Period. Nor is homeopathic medicine appropriate for treating heart disease, cancer, or other serious diseases.

There are gray areas, though. Topical homeopathic remedies like arnica appear to reduce arthritic pain, inflammation, and bruises, and some people swear by a homeopathic remedy made from the herb passionflower to help them sleep better. You may find that a homeopathic remedy works in certain cases, but for something serious you should always continue to rely on mainstream medicine to diagnose a problem and treat diseases.

VITAMIN AND MINERAL SUPPLEMENTS

Almost every day, some new vitamin or supplement promises to be the newest miracle cure. But the science, as we know, is always evolving. One day it's take this; the next day it's don't bother. I have altered my own supplement program recently, and Dr. Andrew Weil has even changed some of his recommendations. Where once he called for 1,000 milligrams of vitamin C daily, now he says 250 milligrams are adequate, since that's all our bodies can assimilate in a day. He's even downgraded his recommendations for vitamin E — once considered a panacea for heart trouble and other ills — from 400 to 800 IUs daily down to a minimum of 80 milligrams of natural mixed tocopherols and tocotrienols (two forms of the nutrient). I used to give the same advice, until I read an important study published in the *Journal of the*

TRUTH

I believe one of the best "vitamin supplements" is eating lots of fruits and vegetables, and they don't always have to be fresh. Frozen is fine; just watch how you handle the packages. When frozen food is allowed to freeze and rethaw, it loses many vitamins. So next time you're in the supermarket, check those containers for signs of thawing. Vegetables like peas or corn should feel loose or break apart easily in the bag — and not feel like a solid chunk of ice. And boxes of spinach and other greens should have their weight evenly distributed, not all lumped to one side. Another tip: think plain. Those fancy sauces not only add to your grocery bill, they can add a lot of fat and sodium to an otherwise healthy serving of veggies. Once you've made your choices, don't waste any time getting them home and into your freezer; they should stay fresh for up to six months.

303

NEWS YOU CAN USE

If you're pregnant, have heavy periods, or have been diagnosed with iron deficiency anemia, your M.D. may prescribe iron supplements. Otherwise, most of us can get all the iron we need from lean red meat, poultry, and veggies like lentils and greens. Iron supplements can interact with some meds and other dietary supplements, and they can aggravate ulcers.

American Medical Association in 2005. It pointed out that taking 400 IUs of vitamin E each day *did nothing* to prevent heart attack or stroke. In patients with vascular disease or diabetes, long-term vitamin E supplementation did not prevent cancer, either, and may even increase the risk for heart failure.

Until recently, it was thought that the mineral selenium was worth taking as a supplement, and I thought so, too. Not only is it an antioxidant, meaning that it prevents oxygen from damaging cells, it was also believed to improve the way the body handles sugar and thought to prevent some complications of diabetes. But the addition of selenium supplements (200 micrograms) has now been associated with an increased risk of diabetes. This discovery was made by a group of researchers who followed nearly twelve hundred people, divided into a selenium or a placebo group, for seven years to see who developed diabetes. More selenium takers developed diabetes than those who took the placebo. The results of this study were published in the *Annals of Internal Medicine* in 2007. I realize discoveries like this can all get complicated. But in terms of selenium, I agree that it's a bad idea to supplement at levels as high as 200 micrograms. What you require in terms of selenium is easily obtainable from your diet. If you take a multivitamin/mineral pill, it already contains some selenium, so you should have yourself covered.

NEWS YOU CAN USE

Used to be, beta-carotene was heralded as an antioxidant miracle. Not anymore. This nutrient, which the body converts to vitamin A, is not recommended for the general public and should not be taken if you're a smoker. Smokers have a greater risk of lung cancer with regular supplementation of beta-carotene.

You don't want to overdo it by taking a separate selenium pill.

Even that trusty multiple vitamin you're probably taking every day is being eyed critically by some researchers. The reason is that like any medicine, taking more than directed can be harmful. Dosages are put on labels for a reason. Keep in mind, too, that many foods, beverages, even over-the-counter medicines are now being plumped up with vitamins and minerals, so you may be megadosing without knowing it.

Recently, researchers at the National Cancer Institute reported that men who pop too many multivitamins a week (more than seven) in the hope of improving their health may in fact be raising their risk of advanced prostate cancer by about 30 percent. This was particularly true in men with a family history of the disease. This was a big study, too: nearly three hundred thousand men were followed over five years to see if there was a link between multivitamin use and prostate cancer. The researchers didn't see any link with overall prostate cancer; the increased risk from overuse of multivitamins was tied to metastatic prostate cancer or cancer that proved fatal. What does this mean to you? Heed the dosage recommendations on the supplement bottle and don't

TRUTH

Lots of herbs are promoted as sexual enhancers, including damiana, gingko, ginseng, maca, and yohimbe. Unfortunately, not enough is scientifically known about these so-called aphrodisiacs, and the claims are usually exaggerated. For conditions like erectile dysfunction, we fortunately have drugs like Viagra, making herbal solutions unnecessary, at least for guys. If you're looking for "natural ways" to improve your sex life, consider trying the following: get plenty of exercise and stay physically active. When you're in shape, you feel better about your body, plus you have more energy — and that includes energy for sex. Also, don't toast your sex life with alcohol. It's a depressant and as such will put a damper on things.

When you have sex, have sex. You don't forget how to ride a bicycle, but you do get rusty at it without practice. The same goes for sex. The more you do it, the more in practice you will be. And always practice safe sex.

go overboard. More is not better, and could be harmful.

While there is debate regarding how worthwhile vitamins and minerals may be, there is no debate about the importance of one supplement: calcium, particularly for menopausal women to protect against osteoporosis. It's important for women to know that their chance of having osteoporosis is as great as breast cancer, ovarian cancer, and uterine cancer combined.

The usual dosage for calcium is 1,000 to 1,500 milligrams. Calcium carbonate and calcium citrate are the most easily absorbed, and most generic supplements are fine. You'll now find all kinds of products fortified with calcium, from aspirin to orange juice. If you have questions, check with your doctor or pharmacist.

You may also want to consider taking an omega-3 supplement. Omega-3 fatty acids, found mostly in fatty fish like salmon, trout, or tuna, benefit the heart if you're healthy or if you are at risk for heart disease. Many fish oil supplements are formulated with omega-3 fats and another type of omega fat, omega-6 fats, present in many vegetable oils.

The case for omega-3s is so strong that the FDA says sellers of food products and supplements that contain two types of omega-3 fatty acids, eicosapentaenoic acid (EPA) and docosahexaenoic acid (DHA), can now tout their health benefits on labels.

Research has shown that these beneficial fats:

- Decrease the risk of sudden death and arrhythmia
- Decrease thrombosis (abnormal blood clotting)
- Lower triglyceride levels
- Retard the growth of atherosclerotic plaque
- Improve your arterial health
- Lower your blood pressure

The advice on dosage is specific. If you have elevated triglycerides, the American

Heart Association says you may need 2 to 4 grams of the omega-3 fatty acids EPA and DHA as a supplement. If you have documented cardiovascular disease, the association recommends about 1 gram of EPA plus DHA per day, preferably from fatty fish. Supplements are an option, too, but talk to your doctor about them. If you don't have heart disease, try to eat fatty fish at least two times a week.

Getting nutrients from food is always preferable to taking supplements, but sometimes that approach isn't feasible. We all lead such busy lives that it can be very difficult for us to get the nutrients we need on a daily basis. We need to look for simple, convenient solutions, and supplements and fortified foods can help fill that bill.

NEWS YOU CAN USE

Eating yellow and green vegetables may be one of the best ways to avoid age-related macular degeneration, a leading cause of blindness in older adults that hampers central vision, according to a study published in the *Archives of Ophthalmology*.

You will want to discuss your own vitamin regimen with your doctor. Although we don't need a lot of each vitamin or mineral, we do need a variety. While the debate rages and the science changes like the wind, we can continue to use vitamin and mineral supplements in a reasonable manner to support health and for those physical conditions they are known to help. I do believe there is more evidence to support the use of vitamin and mineral supplements than not. Again, keep in mind that these supplements can help in moderation, but too much may be toxic.

Here is a daily regimen I am comfortable with:

- A general multivitamin formulated with anti-oxidants (taken once daily with food)
- Calcium: 500 to 1,500 milligrams daily, depending on your age and quality of your diet
- Vitamin D: 200 IU daily for people nineteen to fifty years old; 400 IU daily for those fifty-one to seventy years old; and 600 IU daily for those seventy-one years and older. (An average multivitamin tablet contains 400 IU of vitamin D. Therefore, your daily multivitamin

should help provide the recommended amount of vitamin D.)

- Omega-3 fatty acids: Talk to your doctor about the proper dosage for you, based on your cardiovascular health.

How to Evaluate Supplements

The supplements I've described for you are ones that I frequently recommend to my patients, primarily because enough science is there to support their benefits. There are a slew of other treatments that may improve health, but the data are too preliminary to recommend the therapy. Some make exaggerated claims about curing diseases; others even ask you to skip treatment from your conventional doctor and resort to their unproven therapies instead. Remember — if it sounds too good to be true, it probably is.

Here are some suggestions that can help you evaluate complementary and integrative treatments so that you don't hurt your wallet or your health.

- Be alert to certain words and phrases. Bogus therapies and products are hyped by descriptors such as "satisfaction guaranteed," "miracle cure," or "new discovery." If the product were in fact a cure, it would be widely re-

TRUTH

According to the *Guinness Book of World Records,* an Iowa farmer holds the title for the longest-lasting hiccups, a full sixty years. Hiccups happen when the diaphragm, the muscle that controls our breathing, temporarily goes haywire. Now, unless you're looking for a place in the record books, there are plenty of remedies you can try the next time you get the hiccups. Breathing into a paper bag is one old-fashioned cure. Some doctors think this calms the diaphragm by increasing the amount of carbon dioxide in your bloodstream. Drinking a large glass of water or holding your breath sometimes works the same way. Stimulating the roof of your mouth may also help. You can gently rub a cotton swab there or bend over and try to drink a glass of water upside down. Even if you don't get rid of your hiccups, you'll at least amuse your friends. And if that doesn't work, here's another creative suggestion: plug both ears with your fingers. One almost certain cure is to try any remedy for five minutes; except for rare cases caused by underlying disorders, that's how long it takes for most hiccups to go away on their own.

ported in the media as such and your doctor would prescribe or recommend it. Also, if the manufacturer claims that a product can treat a kitchen-sink range of symptoms or cure or prevent a number of diseases, that's a red flag, too, since no single product can do it all.

- Scour any supplement or health food website for scientific studies rather than testimonials and anecdotes. Many websites promoting these products contain testimonials, or anecdotes from users, but no solid scientific documentation. If the product or therapy has true scientific merit, the manufacturer will publish the scientific evidence in its promotional materials.
- Understand the basics of scientific studies. If you go the extra step and research alternative products in scientific

journals, assess the quality of the research. This is easy to do. Look for the following words and phrases: *clinical study,* which involve studies on humans — not animals; *double-blind,* in which neither the researchers nor the human subjects know who will receive the active treatment and who will receive an inactive substance called a placebo; or *randomized,* in which participants are divided into two groups — one receiv-

TRUTH

Coffee cannot sober you up.

Nor does it rid your system of alcohol, contrary to popular belief. The reason people believe that drinking coffee can reverse the effects of alcohol is that coffee partially reverses the sedating effect of the alcohol. Be a responsible drinker and don't get to the point where you feel you need to sober up. And if you've been drinking, always have a designated driver, someone who hasn't had any alcohol that evening.

ing the standard treatment, another receiving no treatment or a placebo. Also make sure the study is published in a "peer-reviewed" journal, meaning that a watchdog panel of experts reviews the science.

- Be wary of false accusations. One of my favorites is the claim that includes some form of the phrase "what your doctor (or the government) doesn't want you to know." Such conspiracies are rarely true. Basically, the manufacturer is accusing (falsely) the government or the medical profession of suppressing product information that can help people. We may all have objections to organized medicine and federal agencies from time to time, but no one is trying to keep you from learning the truth.

Ideally, any natural supplement you take should work together with medication that has been prescribed by your doctor. The treatments may complement each other; then again, they may not. You need to do your homework before taking any supplement, and again, for your safety tell your doctor everything you're taking — even if your doctor looks at you disapprovingly.

■ ■ ■ ■

There's one final myth involving something so central to our health and longevity that it can go neither unchallenged or unmentioned — and it affects our mental health. Read on to learn how to make each passing year better than the one before.

MYTH #7 . . .

YOU CAN JUST SNAP OUT OF MENTAL ILLNESS

There's a lot to be said for living your life to the fullest, but sometimes there are bumpy detours and side roads. Things happen that you don't expect. You get in bad relationships; someone dies; you lose your job. Those things interfere, and it's not always pretty. We salute those who stoically weather the storms of life or who are serene in the face of great loss or pain. But our attitude is different toward those who resort to therapy or prescription drugs for depression or anxiety; we sometimes see their choice as an admission of weakness, a sign that they can't quite manage things on their own, a failure of will or strength.

We think that people should be able to snap out of depression and anxiety, because we don't recognize that they are treatable illnesses. But in the case of mental health, such attitudes can stand in the way of recognizing when things get off track and when it might be time for measures that help restore joy, energy, and purpose to life.

I learned about the impact mental illness can have on one's life when I was a sophomore at Indiana University and was raped by an intruder who found his way into what I thought was a safe and secure world. The room I shared with my roommate, Sandy, was the fourth door down the hall from the stairway that gave access to the building. The doors to our dorm were supposed to be locked and usually were. Our dorm room had a bolted lock, but that night I left it ajar so that Sandy, who was studying calculus downstairs with a fellow math student, could get back in without awakening me. I had gone to bed early because I had classes the next morning and wanted to get as much sleep as possible.

What happened after I fell asleep is fragmented in my memory like an incomplete jigsaw puzzle, with many missing pieces. Someone was on top of me, an unkempt white man, a knife in his hand. I don't remember even his leaving. I recall taking a shower and, hours later, wandering around the campus in the early morning until the campus police politely deposited me back in my room. The next day, pretending nothing had happened, I picked up where I left off, dutifully going to classes, studying, and living life in suspended animation. There was safety in not thinking, not remembering. Then I broke.

I cried uncontrollably, and at the drop of a hat. I skipped classes. I got fat. Every day I felt trapped — like being in a stainless-steel canister, unable to climb up the slick sides to escape. I settled into a deep depression, never sharing with anyone the trauma that had sent me spiraling downward.

Two years later, during Thanksgiving vacation of my senior year, I ended my self-imposed exile. I blurted out to my parents that I had been raped. My parents' pain was palpable, not only over the horror of what had happened but that they hadn't been able to protect me from it. They did their best to help me heal. My father took me to Chicago to shop and go to the theater. My mother tucked me in at night when I was home. Every gesture helped but drifted away like a breeze the second it was over. I confessed to my dad that I was really depressed and needed to see a psychiatrist. The timing could not have been worse. This was 1971 and mental illness was for crazy people who needed to be locked up. It didn't affect middle-class girls from suburbia. Back then, depression was not something many people

TRUTH

I have always been an animal lover, and at times in my life I have owned horses, dogs, and cats. But my love of pets aside, the science is there that owning a dog and caring for it is good for your health. Studies have found that dog owners age fifty and older visit the doctor less often, have fewer illnesses, and recover more quickly from illnesses than do people without dogs. Having a dog also gives you a reason to take a walk.

The mere physical contact with a dog or other pet can be a source of comfort and may decrease loneliness. Many hospitals and health-care facilities now employ "therapy dogs" that visit patients, who in turn are often more active and responsive during and after the visits. Having a pet may also reduce anxiety, since interacting with it can distract you from stress. I also think pet ownership makes you less selfish, since you have to think about another creature other than yourself. But choose

Truth, *continued*

your pets wisely. There is nothing stress reducing about a dog that chews your favorite chair to bits or barks all night.

confessed to. Confessing cost Missouri senator Thomas Eagleton the nomination for vice president. The press and the American public were horrified, and it was the end of Eagleton's political career.

So this was the backdrop and the reference point for my father's response: "If anyone finds out you've been treated for depression, you'll never get into medical school. This might well keep you from getting in and becoming a doctor." He was probably right. So I just went forward and dealt with the demons of shame, unworthiness, and fear, as they insinuated themselves into my life. I did not go into therapy or seek other help. I continued to let the flow of everyday life — the progression of days and months, waking and sleeping, going to classes, getting into medical school, and finally, graduating — carry me further and further from that awful night. It was not until I was a young surgeon on the staff at the University of Arkansas for Medical Sciences that I would get the help I needed and start to put the pieces of my life back together.

Years later, now married with three children, depression was not so hard to recognize when it struck home again. My husband, Doug, came down with Lyme disease, and he was hit hard. Lyme disease is known to disrupt the central nervous system, causing meningitis, memory loss, inability to concentrate, and depression, among other afflictions.

Doug, a former air force fighter pilot, is a gifted television sports producer (the Emmys in our house belong to him, not me) and is often out of town months at a time to produce major sports events like the Olympics. We are two independent people who happen to be married to each other, and ours is a lifestyle that works for us (though when he is gone, someone invariably asks me how long I've been a single mom!).

Doug has always been — and is — athletic, smart, and a terrifically handsome guy. He started experiencing headaches and muscle pains that eventually gave way to facial paralysis, meningitis, and Guillain-Barré syndrome, a rare inflammatory disorder in which the body's immune system attacks the nerves. Within days, he was paralyzed up to

TRUTH

Psychological problems do not cause inflammatory bowel disease.

Inflammatory bowel disease (IBD) is the term for a group of disorders that cause the intestines to become red and swollen. Two kinds of inflammatory bowel disease are Crohn's disease and ulcerative colitis. Contrary to popular belief, stress, anxiety, or other psychological problems do not cause these illnesses. Most medical experts believe they are triggered by a virus or bacteria that activates an abnormal reaction in the immune system leading to inflammation in the intestines. Stress, however, can *aggravate* the symptoms of abdominal pain and diarrhea associated with IBD, but it does not cause it.

his chest. We were scared.

Thankfully, we found out that his condition was not life-threatening, but soon he began wrestling with its aftermath. This avid mountain biker and international adventure rider was walking with two canes, and the muscles in his thighs and upper arms had withered like an old man's. All the activities he loved were now out of reach. But his physical body wasn't the only thing to betray him. The meningitis took a toll on his brain and his personality.

That he was depressed was brought to my attention in a curious way — from a photograph of the two of us taken at a friend's wedding. There was my husband, sitting at a table, his hair long and unkempt, his face unshaven, his pants baggy, his shirt wrinkled. It was as if I had picked up a guy off the street. One of the ways you can tell someone is depressed is when they stop taking care of their appearance. I was so shocked by the image staring back at me from the photo that I had no choice but to confront him. He denied feeling depressed and, not surprisingly, took a path that people often choose — to look away from the problem and avoid dealing with it. He honestly could not see the difference between himself and everyone around him.

A severe depression like his does not go away on its own, nor can it be waved off with a pep talk. It goes far deeper than that. When a person you live with is depressed, the problem escalates and the entire family is bruised. Doug snapped at the children, he withdrew, and he was no longer affectionate.

TRUTH

Some women become depressed after delivering a baby, and this is termed *postpartum depression* or the *baby blues*. No one knows the exact cause, but it is thought to be related to the complex mix of physical, hormonal, emotional, and psychological changes associated with having a baby. For example, the levels of estrogen and progesterone, the female reproductive hormones, increase by ten times during pregnancy but plummet after delivery, which could explain a new mother's unprovoked crying, irritability, and spikes of elation. Women who undergo a Cesarean delivery are highly prone to postpartum depression. Exactly why, we don't know, but some therapists say that in certain cases Cesarean delivery can cause effects similar to posttraumatic stress syndrome. For some women expecting to give birth by vaginal delivery, having a C-section may bring on frustration, anxiety, or depression. There are ways to prevent or cope with postpartum depression: Ask for help after you get home. Talk about your feelings; suffering alone and in silence will only add to your depression. Your body has just been through an arduous process, so try to sleep as much as possible after giving birth. Follow a healthy diet. The baby blues are usually transient, lasting only a few weeks. If your depression continues to pull you down, talk to your doctor.

He pushed the kids and me away. The real Doug was slipping away from us.

The first step was to have him see his doctor to make sure that the treatment for Lyme disease was on course. The next steps involved seeing a psychologist for therapy and taking antidepressants. The latter proved to be a hurdle. He was against taking any medicines. His attitude was that taking a drug made him a morally weak human being and that he was above it all. I begged him, and after a lot of badgering he relented, albeit begrudgingly. Once on the medication, the Doug I knew slowly reemerged, as the paralyzing veil of depression lifted. He protested that he didn't feel different, and he hated being on a drug with no "finish line" in sight. But that misconception was part of the problem. He expected an antidepressant to make him feel jazzed; he didn't understand that the goal was to get him back on the playing field. Just when I thought he was on track, without telling me, he stopped taking the medicine. Sure enough, the mood swings, the irritability, the low libido all came back. He didn't see any of it. But we did.

We were in a crisis, and I had to be caringly forceful. Basically, one day I said to him, "I won't divorce you because I don't want to do that to the kids, but I can't be your partner anymore. Your depression is affecting our marriage, our family, and our life. You aren't listening to the people who love you. We seem to care more about you than you do."

Doug read the look on my face; he knew my ultimatum was for real. As a family, we were unraveling. He went back on the medication and even heeded my plea to continue with professional help. Little by little, he eased back into normalcy. Therapy was a new experience for him, but it helped him confront the fact that he felt as though his body had betrayed him. He started a strength-training program that left him energized and feeling more in control of his body. Doug began to comprehend that he

TRUTH

Boring jobs can kill you.

Conventional wisdom would have us think that being in charge of a large corporation and making difficult decisions all day would be the ticket to an early grave. But it turns out that this just isn't the case. It's that boring, humdrum job that can actually kill you. So says a study from the University of Texas School of Public Health. Researchers found that workers in undemanding jobs, with little control over what they do, are 35 percent more likely to drop dead in a given ten-year period than workers in more challenging positions. Why? It seems to be the loss of control over your life. Having some control over the decisions in your life helps decrease stress and the natural surge of chemicals that comes with it. What to do about it? Figure out what it is about your job that you hate and then fix it. If your only employment option is being stuck on an assembly line, then find some joy on your breaks or after work. Remedying the boredom is essential.

could reclaim the person he once was. Though at the time the grip of his depression seemed unbreakable, he was eventually able to go off the antidepressant, discontinue therapy, and reconnect with himself and our family.

ANATOMY OF A MYTH

Here is an encouraging, empowering fact to take to heart: mental disorders like depression and anxiety are illnesses, and you are no more responsible for them than you would be if you had diabetes — and if you did have diabetes, you would not hesitate to treat it. Mental health problems are not caused by the person suffering from them, either. Certainly, you need to take responsibility for the thoughts, feelings, and behaviors associated with the problem, but you are not to blame for them. The way I see it, there is a difference between taking responsibility and accepting blame — and it's important to not confuse the two. Mental disorders do not reflect character flaws or signs of moral, emotional, or intellectual weakness. There is no single "cause" for mental illness. A whole nexus of factors is involved — like family history, stress, chronic illness, or brain chemical imbalances — and only some of these are in our control. Depression and anxiety cannot always be ameliorated by simply thinking "positive thoughts" or by "getting hold of oneself." Nor can you always just snap out of them because someone wants you to. Yes, some depression and anxiety, but not all, pass. If they don't, that's when you need professional help. Getting help when you need it will make you stronger. In fact, asking for help is not ever a sign of weakness; it is a sign of strength. If you think you can't get through a particular event, change, or transition in your life without help, you're ahead of the game.

Paying attention to our mental health is just as important to our well-being as is our physical health — maybe more so, since our state of mind inevitably influences how we take care of ourselves. Despite the social stigmas attached to them, mental health problems are neither rare nor unusual. One in five adult Americans will experience a diagnosable mental disorder within their lifetime, according to the National Institute of Mental Health (NIMH). In addition, mental disorders are the leading cause of disability in the United States for people ages fifteen to forty-four. And many people suffer from more than one mental disorder at a given time.

As a Western-trained surgeon, I was taught

the old dogma that the mind and body are separate. But the truth is that the mind and body in both health and sickness are parts of a single whole, and most doctors now recognize this. The brain is an organ just like the heart, liver, or kidneys, and it operates on the same biochemical principles. When we experience any emotion, good or bad, a complex interaction of chemicals and electrical activity goes on inside our cells.

Take stress as a very simple example. The stress that millions of us feel trying to juggle the pressures at home, on the job, with our kids, or over our finances, can flood our bodies with stress hormones: epinephrine, commonly called adrenaline; norepinephrine, and glucocorticoids like cortisol. Epinephrine and cortisol are released by the adrenal glands, tiny organs that sit on top of the kidneys; norepinephrine is released by nerve cells. These chemicals are discharged in the powerful cascade of our "fight / flight" reflex that has governed humans since we ran on the plains and hunted wild animals.

Today, whenever a person is in a challenging, threatening, or stressful situation, the same chemicals are released. They heighten the senses, make the heart pound, and push sugar into the bloodstream for ready energy. They're useful in the short term to mobilize

TRUTH

A growing body of research says happiness is not only a state of mind, it's a state of health. In 2007 I filed a medical report for NBC and MSNBC on the relationship between happiness and health, focusing on two studies. One was at Carnegie Mellon University where researchers found that "happy" subjects exposed to cold and flu viruses were less susceptible to illness than their more negative counterparts. The other study was done in a most unusual place — at Villa Assumpta in Baltimore and at six other convents around the United States. Researchers looked at short autobiographies of 678 nuns. They found that those who used the most "positive" words lived, on average, ten years longer than nuns expressing more negative emotions. One of the sisters, Genevieve Kunkel (who, at the age of one hundred, has never had a major health problem) told me: "If we hope, we cope. If we don't, we mope." Words to live by, indeed.

Without stress, life might be pretty boring. Fortunately, the better you cope with it, the better your "good" HDL cholesterol level is likely to be, according to a study at Oregon State University in Corvallis.

us for action until the threat passes. They are meant to pulse through our system during emergencies, not on a daily basis. But when they do, this can lead to high blood pressure, obesity, and over time, a weakened immune system. Most mental disorders, from depression to anxiety, have their origins in underlying biology and neurochemistry. Some we understand well; others we are just beginning to unravel.

An illness of the mind can also trigger or worsen diseases in the body, which is why we must stop marginalizing mental health problems and put their treatment on par with other chronic illnesses. Depression, for instance, can do more physical damage to someone's health than several long-term diseases, according to a study published in 2007 in *The Lancet*.

Researchers from the World Health Organization studied the physical effects of several illnesses by analyzing data from more than 245,000 people in sixty countries. Their results showed that depression had more health-impairing impact on sufferers than angina, arthritis, asthma, and diabetes. Also, according to the study, after heart disease, depression is expected to become the second-leading cause of "disease burden," a measure of the number of years of complete health lost owing to an illness, by the year 2020. It's a fact, too, that once you have had a heart attack, your risk of dying from cardiovascular disease is higher if you also suffer from depression. People with cancer, diabetes, osteoporosis, and other illnesses have higher odds of experiencing disability or premature death if they are clinically depressed.

NEWS YOU CAN USE

Practice meditation if you have rheumatoid arthritis (RA), an autoimmune disease in which the disease-fighting cells of the immune system attack the joints. In a study published in *Arthritis Care & Research,* RA patients were better able to cope with their disease after learning and practicing meditation for six months.

That's where the vicious cycle begins. People with chronic illnesses are more likely to be depressed, and depressed people are more likely to succumb to chronic illnesses. It's natural to feel depressed when dealing with a chronic, potentially fatal illness, but that alone does not explain depression's damaging effects. Mental illness adversely alters the chemical balance of the body. In patients with diabetes, for example, depression makes the body even less sensitive to insulin, the hormone that processes blood sugar, and thus further aggravates the disease. Fixing a problem in one place, thankfully, can often help in the other.

Understanding Anxiety and Depression

What are some of the major mental disorders? They take many forms, but the two major classifications, as grouped by the NIMH, are mood disorders and anxiety disorders. Of the two, anxiety disorders are the most prevalent mental health problem experienced by adults, affecting nearly forty million people in the United States. While anxiety can mobilize people to get a job done, whether that means meeting a deadline, ending a stormy relationship, or rushing a child to the emergency room, it becomes a problem when it persists too long beyond the initial challenge or threat and life feels out of control. Someone who is extremely anxious may have trouble sleeping, eating, working, enjoying sex, or relaxing.

There are many different forms of anxiety, from phobias to panic attacks to posttraumatic stress syndrome. Because this chapter takes a broad-brush look at anxiety, it is impossible to go into as much detail as I would like to in many important areas of this disorder. A great source for more information is the NIMH website, www.nimh.nih.gov.

Mood disorders include major depressive disorder and bipolar disorder (also called manic depression). There's a difference between these disorders and feeling sad. Every one of us feels "blue" or "down in the dumps" from time to time, and when we talk

TRUTH

A lot of us have trouble with our memory. This happens to me when I am expected at the drop of a hat to spit out my kid's ages. The other day, for example, I said one of my daughters was nineteen and she blurted out that she was twenty-one. Does this mean Alzheimer's disease? No. While forgetting ages, names, appointments, or phone numbers is normal, people with Alzheimer's forget this information more often and have trouble remembering it later. They also have trouble remembering what common items are. Someone with plain old forgetfulness might forget where he left his keys, but someone with Alzheimer's might look at the keys and say, "What are these?" If you're worried about memory lapses in yourself or someone you love, it's best to visit a doctor to determine the cause of the symptoms.

to close friends, we often use the word *depressed* to refer to an intense feeling of discouragement or sadness tied to a specific event in our lives. Bad days, unexpected outcomes, and even failures are facts of life, as is feeling "down" about them. So is sadness triggered by a painful or life-changing event or loss — a divorce in the family, a broken heart, death, or even relocating to a new town. Feeling sad now and then or, after a major loss, for a longer period of time, is part and parcel of the human condition. Such depression, however, usually does not last. It comes, you figure it out, and move on.

Depression in the clinical sense is quite different. It shows no signs of letting up and it is incapacitating. Clinical depression, or "major depression," affects every part of us

NEWS YOU CAN USE

For a better night's sleep, disengage all your electronic gadgets an hour before bedtime. These include your computer, BlackBerry, and cell phone. If your computer is in your bedroom, turn off the screen, too. The ambient light can interfere with sleep.

— how we think, feel, and act, both physically and emotionally — and it goes beyond merely having the blues. The line has crossed from normal mood swings to feelings of hopelessness or pessimism. People suffering from clinical depression may experience irritability, restlessness, and helplessness. They may feel like they are dragging themselves through the day. They may feel worthless and unmotivated. All the things that used to be pleasurable are no longer worth the effort. Making decisions, concentrating, and remembering seem difficult or impossible. In addition, major depression may be accompanied by severely disturbed sleep patterns and loss of appetite. Others may put on weight and sleep much of the day when depressed. They may also be drawn to thoughts of suicide as relief from their depression.

I'm sure you've probably heard of bipolar disorder. Not nearly as prevalent as other forms of depressive disorders, bipolar disorder is characterized by severe and unpredictable mood swings. Moods are certainly part of life and are often effective in causing us to make life-enhancing decisions and changes. The person with bipolar disorder swings between severe highs (mania) and lows (depression). When in the low cycle, someone can have any or all of the symptoms of major depression. When in the manic cycle, he or she may be overactive, overtalkative, and have a great deal of energy. There is a side to this disorder that can make treatment a real challenge: a creative person battling the disorder may be creative only during the manic phase (some of our most famous stand-up comedians are like this). Treating the mania can dampen that creative spirit, and sometimes patients hate that. But if your doctor understands this, treatment can be tailored so that creative genius can remain intact and flourish.

THE BRIGHT SIDE OF THE PICTURE: GETTING RELIEF

Fortunately, there are so many treatments now available, that depression and anxiety can be effectively and expeditiously nipped in the bud — which means you can bounce back and return to productive living in no time at all.

If you find yourself unable to shake a gloomy mood, experiencing severe highs and lows, or habitually feeling a deep persistent fear or anxiety — and you know this is not like you or normal — you must ask for help. Monitoring your own mental health should be as important and as routine as seeing your doctor and getting your annual checkup. If you are concerned about your mental state and behavior, you should feel as justified in seeking help as you would for going for tests because you found a suspicious lump or because you're experiencing physical pain that doesn't seem to go away.

If you feel like you are suffering from an anxiety or a mood disorder, the first step is to consult your doctor and have a physical examination to rule out any physical causes of your feelings. Remember, conditions such as an underactive thyroid, low blood sugar, diabetes, heart disease, arthritis, or even bowel disorders can cause depression. So can some medications, such as oral contraceptives and corticosteroids. If a clinical illness is ruled out, your doctor will be able to help you find a reliable therapist, psychologist, or psychiatrist. Depending on your diagnosis, you may be prescribed medication or one of several forms of psychotherapy known to be effective. The basic strategy for the treatment of a mood or anxiety disorder is an integrated treatment approach that often involves relieving symptoms with medication, under your doctor's guidance, and seeking professional help from a qualified mental health counselor, psychologist, or psychiatrist.

TRUTH

Chocolate does wonders for your body.

I have a friend who says chocolate is so wonderful that it should be its own food group. Something I know for sure about chocolate is that it contains natural compounds with some rather intriguing properties. One compound makes blood platelets less likely to stick together and cause abnormal clots. This helps blood flow, promotes normal clotting, and improves circulation. Another compound is a stimulant called phenylethylamine, dubbed the "love chemical," which promotes the euphoria that comes with falling in love. The darker the chocolate, the better, since dark chocolate has the most healthful properties. Look for chocolate with at least 70 percent cocoa in it for the best benefit . . . and enjoy a little every day.

Therapy

At a time in my thirties, when life wasn't quite working for me — I was recovering from a divorce, adjusting to a new job and a new city, and facing economic pressure — I decided to see a therapist for counseling. I hesitated at first. I saw it not only as a sign of weakness but as a type of self-indulgence, too, a New York City type of thing out of a Woody Allen movie: lying on a couch, once a week, for years on end, talking about yourself, getting nowhere. Of course, I was dead wrong.

I came to realize that an important first step in getting better was to admit that I could not go it alone during that period of my life. I was trying to be everything for everyone else, and in doing so I felt empty and hollow. How could I expect other people to like me if I didn't like myself? So I began a journey of self-discovery and renewal through therapy. I had to get help for myself. And I discovered that this was not a sign of weakness but of resilience.

About once a week, I visited a therapist and found it was like having a new friend in my life, someone I could talk to about what was really going on in my head and get advice in return. During therapy, my therapist told me something that would help turn my life around, and it stayed with me forever: "What the world thinks of you is none of your business." This wisdom helped me stop trying to please everyone and take care of

TRUTH

Doing good deeds does a body good.

Volunteering for a cause you believe in, helping a neighbor in need, donating money — these acts of altruism come back to you in positive ways. There's a growing body of data showing that people who give more to their friends and family than they receive — whether the gift was in the form of money, food, resources, or time — report feeling healthier than others, even when activity levels are factored in. Clearly, one of the best ways to stay healthy is to be kind to others.

myself first.

If you are healthy and emotionally stable, you'll be able to give to those around you. Not worrying about getting affirmation from the multitudes frees you to be yourself and walk your own path. Counseling eventually peeled away layer after layer of self-doubt, helping me recognize the parts of myself that were valuable and worthy, and I credit it with my successful turnaround.

For those who take on the work of under-going therapy, the options are growing. Immediate results can be gained through short-term counseling (ten to twenty weeks) with cognitive and behavioral therapy, which teach coping skills. Psychodynamic therapy, which explores issues and traumas of the past, can bring to the surface deeply rooted conflicts behind a problem.

It doesn't really matter how much time you invest or the approach you take. What is important is to become healthy again. Mental health disorders are poor company and can haunt you all your life if left untreated. They should not be ignored.

And do your homework. It's critical to get psychiatric help from someone who is well-versed in the disorder from which you are suffering.

Lifestyle Measures

Don't underestimate the effect of your lifestyle on your moods and feelings. The lifestyle you choose can help counteract symptoms while you start treatment. I think it's a good idea to take stock of your daily habits and patterns to see what might be adding to your anxiety or depression and what you might be able to change in your lifestyle — so consider keeping a food and activity diary. Chart your mood. Are there any patterns? Are you getting enough sleep? Keep your notes for a month and share them with your doctor and therapist. You may be surprised how little changes in your life can have big effects on how you feel. In addition, consider the following tips:

- Talk it out. Don't do what I did back when I was in college and not confide in anyone. Join a support group, or tell your friends about your moods or anxieties. Both approaches let you express your feelings and thus lessen them, and both are good ways to let others help you achieve a sense of perspective regarding what is troubling you.

- Look into relaxation techniques and meditation; these are some of the best ways to lighten your load and reduce anxiety and depression. If you don't think you have enough time, then carve out fifteen minutes at the end of the day when no one is around to bother you. Yoga and other mind–body forms of exercise are effective at reducing anxiety, relieving stress, and lifting depression. Yoga classes are available in almost all communities, fitness centers, or on DVDs that you can find easily in your library or local video store.

- Try to maintain a healthy diet. You've heard it all before, but eat a lot of fruits and vegetables; they're essential to keeping your body and brain fit. Consider adding omega-3 fatty acids to your diet — known to naturally help alleviate depression since they appear to help boost serotonin in the brain. You can get them from cold-water fish such as tuna, salmon, or mackerel.

- Say good-bye to alcohol (except for that occasional glass of red wine). Eliminating alcoholic beverages from your diet can help you counteract the symptoms of depression, since alcohol is a depressant itself and interferes with sleep. If you are taking tranquilizers for anxiety, you must abstain from alcohol because they interact and can be more toxic to your system than either one can alone. Alcohol and most medicines are also metabolized by the liver and combining them can cause liver damage over time.

- Exercise, and if you have the option, get some exercise outdoors, even if that means just walking around the block. Exercise releases endorphins, nature's "joy" chemicals, which relax and calm the body and give you a sense of well-being. Exercise also relieves stress and anxiety and can diminish depression.

- Get some sunlight. Some depressive moods are triggered by a lack of sunshine. In fact, seasonal affective disorder (SAD), a type of depression affecting about thirteen million Americans, seems to strike people during the fall and winter and disappears during summer. A little time in the sunlight helps increase serotonin levels in the brain. SAD can also be treated with the anti-depressant Wellbutrin.

- Have a reason to get out of bed in the morning. If you don't have anyone to live for, there are plenty of people out in the world who need someone. Get out of bed, put on your clothes, eat breakfast, and go volunteer — at a local shelter, the hospital, or for your favorite charity. There's always something to do.

- Learn how to breathe correctly. Breathing is the window to good health, both physical and mental. Most of us do it wrong. We breathe quickly and shallowly, and in times of stress we even hold our breath. Retraining yourself to breathe properly is effective for reducing the physical effects of anxiety, in particular. When severely anxious or in the throes of a panic attack, some people hyperventilate, which manifests in shallow, tense breathing; chest pain; dizziness; even fainting. Practice measured, controlled breathing. Begin breathing from your abdomen. Then slow your breaths by counting to four with each inhale and exhale. Let your abdomen expand each time you breathe in and contract each time you breathe out.

Prescription Medicine

We have learned so much about the neurochemistry of the brain over the past couple of decades, and the pharmaceutical industry has responded with medications for a variety of disorders. The medicines I'll discuss here are just some of those available today. Breakthroughs occur daily. For my husband, an antidepressant was part of his recovery, and for millions of others these drugs have been lifesaving. But you shouldn't forget that they are powerful medicines, they don't work for everyone, and they can have real side effects.

Make sure your doctor knows all about your illness and chooses the medicine carefully in conjunction with you, and that you keep in touch regarding any side effects. Personally, I believe these medicines should always be used together with therapy. Talking about your problems, no matter how trivial they may seem, can be just as important as taking a pill.

Medications for mood or anxiety disorders are designed to restore depleted neurotransmitters and bring them back into balance. If you are suffering from an anxiety disorder, your doctor may prescribe a tranquilizer, and counseling may also be recommended. Tranquilizers belonging to the benzodiazepine group (including Valium, Xanax, Librium, Klonopin, and Ativan) are the most commonly prescribed for anxiety. They differ mainly in duration of effect, but their clinical effects are nearly identical. They have a calming or sedative effect and work as central nervous system depressants. A different type of antianxiety medication often prescribed is BuSpar. It influences the activity of certain neurotransmitters that are thought to play a role in anxiety disorders. Antidepressants are often used to treat anxiety as well. Tranquilizers are potent and can be addictive, so they need to be taken with care, respect, and caution.

The most common antidepressants for

TRUTH

Sleep deprivation brings on the blues.

Lack of sleep and poor sleep quality make the body churn out excess cortisol, a stress hormone. Too much cortisol hanging around in your body can impair memory, elevate blood pressure, sap your immune system, and bring on depression. Better sleep helps ameliorate this imbalance. So chase away the blues by getting on a regular sleep schedule and sticking to it.

treating depression and other mood disorders are selective serotonin reuptake inhibitors, or SSRIs; serotonin-norepinephrine reuptake inhibitors, or SNRIs; and norepinephrine and dopamine reuptake inhibitors, or NDRIs. The effectiveness of SSRIs such as Lexapro, Zoloft, Paxil, and Prozac hinges on the drugs' selectivity for serotonin, a chemical in the body that triggers the pleasure center. Serotonin is vitally important to your brain, where it helps regulate activities from eating and sleeping to pain and moods. SSRIs keep serotonin from being reabsorbed quickly into nerve cells when it is produced, raising the levels of available serotonin in your brain. SNRIs increase the levels of not only serotonin but also norepinephrine by inhibiting the reabsorption of both into cells in the brain. Effexor and Cymbalta are two widely prescribed SNRIs. The only NDRI currently approved is Wellbutrin; it was developed to balance the levels of the chemicals dopamine and norepinephrine in the body. Wellbutrin is also sold as Zyban, a drug to help people quit smoking.

Bipolar disorder has been effectively treated with lithium as a first-line treatment for stabilizing mood. Now therapy is being fine-tuned with medications like anticonvul-

TRUTH

Studies show that smokers do seem more prone to depression, although medical experts aren't sure why. They speculate that nicotine (even though it has mood-elevating properties) and other tobacco by-products interfere with the uptake of brain chemicals. This makes sense when you consider that an antidepressant like Wellbutrin helps balance brain chemicals and is also marketed as a smoking-cessation drug called Zyban.

sants (which regulate moods) and antidepressants. A medication called Seroquel treats both the manic and depressive episodes of bipolar disorder by regulating the balance of chemicals in the brain.

Sometimes researchers find new uses for older drugs. Such is the case with the antiestrogen drug tamoxifen, best known as a treatment for breast cancer. It has been found in an NIMH study to dramatically reduce the symptoms of the manic phase of bipolar disorder — and does so faster than many of the standard drugs for this illness. Tamoxifen appears to block a cell-regulating enzyme that is thought to be overactive during the manic phase of bipolar disorder. Nonetheless, there is still a great deal of research to be done on tamoxifen as an antidepressant before it joins the rank of treatments for bipolar disorder.

Sometimes, people don't always respond to the medication they've been prescribed. If this happens to you, you may decide to stop taking the medicine altogether. You may also find relief by switching to another drug or sometimes by taking a combination of medications. Until a few years ago, doctors didn't know whether switching to a different drug or using combination therapy would work. But results from a large-scale government-funded study called the STAR*D (Sequenced Treatment Alternatives to Relieve Depression) trial found that when people who didn't do well on one antidepressant changed to another one, their symptoms diminished. In another part of the study, 30 percent of 565 patients who supplemented one antidepressant with another recovered from their depression.

So if you're taking an antidepressant but

not feeling better, hang in there. Talk to your doctor, take someone with you to your appointment, and take notes. There may not be a simple fix right away. But medication combined with therapy and a long-term partnership with your doctor is the best approach for tackling these issues.

Whatever the situation, it is important to take your medication until your doctor helps wean you off it. Sometimes, you might rationalize, "I feel fine. I'm well. I don't need these pills anymore." Abandoning medication before your doctor thinks prudent may trigger some serious side effects and also leave you right where you started. If you abruptly stop taking an antidepressant, you might even have withdrawal symptoms. For many people, these are not symptoms they had before, whether it's anxiety or depression but rather symptoms they describe as being worse than the original problem. Withdrawal symptoms are one reason why some people report having bad experiences with these medications. In many cases, the side effects can be minimized if the drugs are tapered off slowly.

Why? Well, one factor is something called the drug's half-life — how long the medicine stays in your body. Paxil, a popular antidepressant, has one of the shortest half-lives,

TRUTH

Over-the-counter painkillers work best before the pain really kicks in.

Being in pain is depressing, and depression causes and intensifies pain. According to the *Harvard Health Letter,* people with chronic pain have three times the average risk of developing psychiatric symptoms — usually mood or anxiety disorders — and depressed patients have three times the average risk of developing chronic pain. If you suffer from pain, even if it is acute pain from an injury or surgery, do not let your pain get out of control. Talk to your doctor about appropriate over-the-counter (OTC) or prescription painkillers or options such as physical therapy, chiropractic medicine, acupuncture, and relaxation techniques. These can complement any other treatment you opt for.

Another move you can make to head off and manage pain, especially if you're active, is to take some ibuprofen or another anti-inflammatory drug before you exercise. Usually the medication keeps the pain from flaring up. If you can anticipate

which means once you stop taking the drug, or even miss a dose, it washes out of the body so quickly that it can cause a jolt to your nervous system. In contrast, Prozac remains in the system longer and is therefore less likely to cause severe withdrawal symptoms.

Withdrawal affects some people more than others, but we don't know why. So do not discontinue a drug without your doctor's knowing about it. And then be prepared for the fact that it may take a while to wean yourself off it.

THOUGHTS OF SUICIDE

At tough times in our lives, most of us have thought about what life would be like without us. Would our pain go away? Would people be better off without us? Fortunately, for most of us, these thoughts are fleeting. We realize that suicide is a permanent solution to a temporary problem.

Persistent thoughts of suicide are a red-flag warning that something is very wrong. If you find yourself drawn to thoughts of suicide, you should seek immediate professional help and/or call a suicide hotline in your community. Depending on what city you live in, a suicide hotline will know where to send you. I am a big believer in peer-trained suicide hotlines. They save lives.

If you know someone is contemplating suicide or even casually mentioning the subject, take it and him or her seriously. Encourage that person to call a hotline and seek help. Suicidal feelings can dissipate once you receive adequate treatment for your depression, anxiety, or other issues.

HELPING THOSE YOU LOVE

From my own experience and dealing with my husband's depression, I can tell you that someone else's depression or anxiety can affect you. There is a ripple effect that goes

TRUTH

Sex is good for your brain.

Sex is pleasurable, and great sex is even more pleasurable. Sex is a way of sharing intimacy. Safe sex is also good for your mental health. Sex releases an assortment of beneficial chemicals in the body to produce a natural euphoria. In addition, satisfying sex leads to better communication and strengthens the bonds between two people, and these can be hedges against depression triggered by relationship issues. So go on and do it.

through the entire family, the workplace, and even the community. When mental illness happens to a loved one, it isn't only that person's problem; it's yours, too. Here are some suggestions that may help you if a loved one is depressed or suffering anxiety.

- Don't try to be a Mr. or Ms. Fix-it. You can't cure someone's depression or anxiety, but you can encourage that person to seek help.

- Recognize that like many illnesses — physical or otherwise — there will be ups and downs in recovery. Don't think it is because someone isn't trying hard enough or that you're not doing all you can. The nature of recovery is often "two steps forward, one step back."
- Understand that you may be pushed away over and over again. Many people who are depressed purposely isolate themselves from others because they know they are unduly causing hurt and will do anything to prevent this from happening, even if it means shutting

TRUTH

Worry and stress won't turn your hair gray.

You can't blame your gray hair on your demanding boss, dwindling checking account, or the antics of your kids. Pigment-producing cells called melanocytes are genetically programmed to stop manufacturing hair pigment at a certain age, regardless of how much stress you have in your life.

TRUTH

You're never too old to start exercising.

If you didn't work out when you were younger, could it be dangerous to start now? Not at all. In a Tufts University study, frail nursing-home residents whose ages ranged from seventy-two to ninety-eight started a strength-training program, and after just ten weeks they improved their muscle strength, ability to climb stairs, and walking speed. Even if you have a chronic disease, exercise is good for you. Some of the greatest benefits are seen in people with arthritis. Exercise reduces pain, plus increases range of motion, strength, and mobility. I don't mean to imply that you can jump right into exercising, regardless of your health. Anyone with an existing illness or multiple risk factors for a disease should check with a physician and start slowly.

out people they love.

- Realize that the depression or the anxiety is the enemy, not your spouse or loved one. These illnesses are like intruders that have stealthily encroached upon your life. The more you are able to look upon them as an "it," the better you'll be able to cope and support the healing process.

- Don't take the person's behavior personally, even if he or she is verbally abusive. If your loved one is irritable, mean, or rejecting, this is typically the depression or the anxiety talking — not the person. Often when people who are depressed or anxious lash out in anger, it's because they are mad at themselves and frustrated with how they feel.
- Provide patience, support, encouragement, and assistance, but do not make your loved one feel totally helpless or inadequate. She needs to take responsibility for getting help and counseling. At the same time, let her know it's the depression or anxiety you're upset with, not her.
- If your loved one is resistant to seeking help, consider asking someone else to intervene. This could be a close relative, a friend, your family doctor, or a member of the clergy. Somewhere along the line, if enough people say, "We are concerned about you," this can

be just the catalyst needed for your loved one to get help.

- Get counseling yourself, if joint counseling is not in the cards. Therapy is helpful in addressing the issues faced by a spouse, partner, or caregiver. Being around someone who is depressed or anxious or otherwise mentally unstable can interfere with your ability to function productively and constructively in your life. If you feel chronically unhappy or unable to cope with the situation, by all means seek help. You are only as good a caregiver to someone else as you are to yourself.

Believing that you or a loved one is worthy of saving, getting help, and changing is the beginning of getting better. We do not snap out of clinical mental disorders; we need help. Taking care of your mental health is not an act of weakness or an admission of failure but a positive, restorative step — and can be the renewed beginning of a better life.

TODAY'S GIFT

As I sit finishing this book, I glance at a piece of paper on my desk. It bears the familiar logo of the American Medical Association. The logo is a serpent coiled around a staff. A strange symbol for medicine, you might say. Stranger yet, it is one that can be traced back to Greek mythology. There is irony in this — don't you think? — with modern medicine swirling in so many myths. The staff belongs to Asclepius, the Greek god of medicine, whose daughter was Hygeia, the Greek goddess of health, and from which the word *hygiene* comes. The ancient Greeks told the story of how sick Greeks prayed for their health at temples dedicated to Asclepius. The sick would sleep in his temples, hoping that Asclepius would visit in a dream and cure them. Asclepius was often portrayed as a bearded man who held a staff encircled by a snake, so priests placed nonpoisonous snakes in the temples to slither about the sick as they slumbered. Hygeia was responsible for maintaining the temples containing these snakes. Like her father, she kept a pet snake and was usually depicted with a serpent and bowl in her hand. In fact, the bowl of Hygeia is a symbol of the pharmacy profession. While Asclepius more directly represented healing, Hygeia represented the prevention of sickness and the continuation of good health.

What we do as doctors can be traced back to the traditions of Asclepius — no, not the snakes but the focus on the physician as hero or rescuer who restores health by treating disease. What we want our patients to do, in partnership with us, can be traced back to the tradition of Hygeia, in which health springs from living wisely. Both traditions remind us that the physician is a healer and that the self-responsibility we have as patients is an integral contribution to the treatment and to the healing we bring. This is a lesson we all need to learn and remember.

Myths, whether ancient or modern day, are instructive and meant to guide us and open our eyes to truth. Using the myths and truths in this book, I hope you have gained information to make the health decisions that will benefit you the most. Personal health can be vast and daunting to most of us, and it is not

CREATE A HEALTH DIARY

I encourage you to do something that I do, and that is keep a health diary. Mine includes who in my family has had breast cancer, colon cancer, and anything else I know about — not just so I can tell my doctor and take better care of myself but also for my children. I want them to know as much as they can about the health of their family so they can protect themselves and take care of their health in the future.

To get started, use a notebook and add to it as you find out more about which relatives had what. Or use your word-processing software to create an electronic record. Your diary should also record treatments or medications that have worked or failed for you or a family member in the past. Record, or tuck in the notebook, copies of test results you've had over the years, and keep them in a sacred place in your home. I take those big manilla envelopes and write MEDICAL on them and throw everything for that year in them. Your system doesn't have to be elaborate; mine sure isn't.

Create a Health Diary, *continued*

Because my eldest daughter, Kate, is adopted, I am often asked by other adoptees, "How can I know what my family history is if I'm adopted?" In that case, I tell them to live their lives as if heart disease and cancer ran in their families, because in many families these diseases do. This means doing the obvious and the humdrum: watching what you eat, exercising, and not smoking. Another course of action is to opt for genetic testing, although it is not foolproof, the technology is in its infancy, and it is expensive. Some people want to do this; others don't care to know. At times it might be the responsible thing to do, particularly if your family history might be suspect.

While I'm curious about what a genetic test might say about me, what would I change if I found something out? I'm fifty-five now — I can't undo all the pizzas I've eaten or the days of exercise I've missed — and I'm doing pretty well as long as my plot at the cemetery is still empty. The blessing in my life is that I've watched how my parents have aged, and this has been a good genetic road map for me. As for

Kate, one of her Christmas presents this year will be the offer of a genetic profile. Okay, it's not something you can rip a shiny ribbon off with abandon and the technology is far from perfect, but it might help usher in the gift of a healthy lifetime. She is twenty-one; she can opt in or opt out, but this is something I'm going to put under the Christmas tree, even though I've raised her to assume that many diseases in life are avoidable, never mind genetics.

friendly territory for the uninformed. One of the best ways to improve the quality and quantity of your life is by being well educated and staying proactive. The more you know, the more control you will have over your life and the course of any treatment you might need. Here are a few ideas on taking good care of yourself as you move forward through your life.

A PERSONAL PLAN FOR STAYING HEALTHY

Because of what you know about yourself, you can take the necessary steps to make sure serious diseases don't sneak up on you or, if you have been diagnosed with something, that it doesn't get worse or progress too rapidly. A positive step in that direction is examining how you live day by day in these six areas:

1. What you eat
2. What you weigh
3. How much you move
4. Whether you smoke
5. How much alcohol you drink
6. How much stress you carry

It's a fairly long list, but I bet you don't even have to worry about all six areas. You probably have just two or three areas in your life that can use additional work, but any one of them might mean a longer, healthier life.

Your Daily Bread

Perhaps you need to let fruits and vegetables dominate your diet; this can be an opportunity to become as healthy as you can be. If you go to a third-world country, where people really rely on grains and vegetables, you'll find that the inhabitants don't have cancer, they don't have heart disease, and they don't have strokes. But we do because we eat all this junk — processed foods and lots of trans fats and saturated fats.

Tweaking your diet might mean making a small change, like vowing to eat breakfast, but it's one that pays big health dividends in the end. Medical evidence says breakfast eaters consume more vitamins and minerals and less cholesterol and fat; they feel more energetic, have greater concentration, and can keep their weight in check. So no matter how rushed you are in the morning, make it a point to eat breakfast, even if you have to eat it in your car.

A Healthy Weight for You

Perhaps you need to review your calorie intake and lose weight. Determine what your ideal weight is and plan how you can get to it through proper diet and exercise. If you need help with this endeavor (and most of us do), consult a nutritionist. There are many reputable meal plans that may help you with the challenge of losing weight.

Move It or Lose It

If you're resistant to exercise, maybe it's time to make it a part of your life. If you're feeling overwhelmed by the prospect of adding exercise to your already hectic life, and if you are feeling defeated by all the years of inactivity you've already accumulated, don't say, "Oh well, I've lost the battle." Any movement you add to your daily routine at any age will help maintain your health. Cleaning your home burns more than 300 calories an hour (that's a bigger expenditure than brisk walking brings), and fast dancing uses up nearly 400 calories! The research is clear — nothing improves life and life expectancy more than exercise.

Don't Smoke!

I can't say it enough: give up smoking. It has a domino effect on many life-shortening diseases, tumbling one defense after another in an overwhelming defeat of good health.

Do All Things in Moderation, Especially Drinking

Keep your alcohol consumption in the moderate range, if you drink, and don't be like a patient I once had who kept claiming he was "overserved." Moderate means no more than one drink a day if you're a woman, no more than two drinks a day if you're a man.

Keep Stress Under Your Control

Most likely you are already taking some measures to kick stress to the curb. But, if not, take a walk, do relaxation exercises, work out, hang out with your friends more often, enjoy a funny movie, dance around your living room — whatever brings you pleasure. And take time for yourself. Doing all or any of these will ease stress and allow you to reserve the emotional energy you need and deserve. And if you're doing all of this already, great, keep it up!

GET STARTED NOW

Here is a simple way to start this process. Review the six areas that impact your health on page 241, or think of some others that apply to you, which may not appear on my list. Pick out three that are of the utmost concern to you. Record them in a notebook or on your computer, and then itemize your specific goals for each of the areas chosen. Here are some examples:

Get more energy.
Eat less red meat and more vegetables.
Enjoy a restful sleep.
Achieve a weight I look and feel good in.
Get glowing skin.
Have no fear of going to the doctor.
Keep a great attitude if I get sick.
Take more time to relax and have fun.
Make exercise a habit.
Live well into my eighties.
Stay well.

The more you are able to be clear about what you want, the better your chances are of moving toward it and then achieving it.

Now, under each goal, record some strategies you can use to create change and accomplish your desired outcomes, and make sure they're quantifiable, doable, realistic, and manageable. For example:

Eat four servings of vegetables each day.
Exercise three hours this week.
Call the doctor today and schedule my annual checkup.
Complete a smoking-cessation class.
Limit my alcohol intake to two drinks on the weekend.

Don't say "I will diet and exercise my way to a size 2" when the smallest you've ever been is a size 8. This is unrealistic and unhealthy, and it sets the stage for possible failure. Make sure your strategies are achievable, and you will succeed.

WHAT DO I DO?

I wish I had a better routine for being more physically active. I, too, fall into the "I don't have time today" trap. To resolve my exercise dilemma, I try to ride my horse at 7 A.M. because I know the world isn't expecting anything of me then. Riding makes for good exercise, despite what it looks like to the uninformed eye. Even so, I feel like I'm sneaking away to do this, as if I were having an affair, and I feel like I'm cheating my family and my employer when I do it.

Like many of you, I'm hard-pressed to find ways to take care of myself in this relentless modern world where seemingly time just disappears. I mistakenly equate taking time for myself to exercise as doing something "wrong" or "bad" as it takes time away from my roles as wife, mother, folder of laundry, doctor, and medical correspondent. Women so often have lives that begin and end with putting the needs of others first. But someone who always puts herself last is not, and cannot be, a good role model for anyone.

Self-denial of health doesn't do anybody any good. In fact, you have to take care of yourself as if your life depended on it, because it does.

What else do I focus on when trying to take better care of myself? My posture is one thing. This might sound silly, but I like it when I feel as though I'm a little longer in the middle. I don't like it when my middle collapses in a slouch. And as a doctor, I know poor posture not only looks unattractive, it also causes aches, pains, poor mobility, stiffness, and tight breathing. How? Slouching puts pressure on your vertebrae, ultimately causing the discs to become compressed and making you vulnerable to back pain. Pelvic muscles go slack, which makes it even harder to support a well-aligned stance, especially as you get older. Nerves in your neck are pinched, too, tightening the muscles there and causing tension headaches. Good posture, on the other hand, makes you feel good. Your muscles are more limber, and you have better mobility and less tension in your upper body. Your back and legs are relaxed; your spine feels longer. And the physiological boost carries over to a sense of psychological well-being. In addition, the way you stand tells people volumes about who you are. Self-assured people walk tall and have a commanding presence when they enter a room — a presence that is both comfortable and confident.

I want to take better care of my feet, too. Think about it: we demand a great deal of our feet and often give them very little in return, yet they carry us everywhere. I always wrap mine in good socks and make sure my feet can take me on good walks. We owe our feet the best possible care as we pound toward our goals and dreams in life.

Modifying your lifestyle isn't meant to be an austerity program but a way of integrating healthy changes you can live with into a life you can enjoy. This is an approach to living that I learned from my parents. My father, at age eighty-four, is sharp as a tack. Back in the fifties, he was a smoker, like practically everyone after World War II, even young doctors. One day, though, he attended a medical meeting at which the surgeon general gave his report showing the link between cigarettes and cancer. Once he saw the science attached to this, my father said, "That's it," and threw away his cigarettes. He met change with change and just went cold turkey. At the same time, he fell in love with jelly beans and kept them around so he could put something in his mouth.

Everything in moderation — that's how my parents live. They aren't vegetarians. They don't abuse alcohol. They enjoy a good bowl of ice cream. They taught me by their example to indulge when the time is right, to diversify. And so I sprinkle the not-so-good-for-you stuff throughout my diet. Yes, I enjoy pizza every now and then with my husband and kids, and on occasion, I like to sip a margarita. It's a lot like investing money. You wouldn't put all your money in one stock — you diversify. So do the same with your food — diversify. Have a sound basic diet and then enjoy some indulgences. It just makes sense.

But here's the rub: we Americans love extremes, and we forget that there are off switches. If we have a bowl of ice cream, we want to eat the whole quart. Then we decide we won't ever eat ice cream again. I think you set yourself up for failure when you do that. There is no secret to a long, healthy life. If there is, it's the secret of moderation. It is this "secret" I bring to my tomorrows, as I look forward to the next fifty years.

LIVING WITH ILLNESS — AND LIVING DESPITE OF IT

Some of you may be dealing with a disease, and it's too much to try to think past it, at least right now. Many years ago, my father-in-law was diagnosed with diabetes. Sure, it was a shock — he'd never been sick a day in his life. Suddenly his zero handicap golf game was suffering, because he had trouble seeing the ball. At first, he didn't like all the changes his doctor said he'd have to make. He started seeing his golf game, business trips, and social life taking a nosedive. But then he saw the silver lining. He refused to accept diabetes as a disease and saw it as a way to improve the quality of his life. He dropped more than forty pounds, began a regular exercise program, and made a game out of which foods could be exchanged for others. He was able to turn diabetes into something productive. This is the way it can be for many people.

Sometimes the lesson of an illness reaches beyond lifestyle change and speaks to another kind of truth. My friend, colleague, and correspondent from the *Today* show, Hoda Kotb, went public some time ago with her breast cancer. Here was someone who at age forty-three was the picture of health. She ate fruit, she jogged, she hardly ever had a cocktail. One day she was fine; the next she was a cancer patient with three lumps in her breast.

The hard moments of life sometimes bestow upon us blessings we would not have imagined. As Hoda told an interviewer, "I do think cancer gave me the gift of being fearless. Cancer gave me the headline, 'You can't scare me.' That takeaway was the biggest thing I've ever gotten." The things in life you think would scare you — like losing all your money or going through a divorce — well, they don't anymore. Adversity makes us brave. Hoda is taking this message to others and using her experience to touch lives.

People like Hoda and my father-in-law, when thrown off balance with a diagnosis, use it as an impetus to change their lives. This is important — finding ways of using your experience to make constructive changes in your life can have a positive impact on how your disease progresses. But more than that, just deciding that there will be another morning to wake up to can be healing and empowering.

WHAT I WANT FOR YOU

In my family we have a tradition that takes on greater meaning with each passing day and makes life all the more meaningful. It was around midday one weekend not too long ago and I was sweeping my kitchen floor. My daughter Rachel called me from Burlington, Vermont. She was walking past a church and from inside, the lilting, familiar chords of Johann Pachelbel's Canon in D gently infused the streets. "This is today's gift," she told me.

One day my son, Charlie, and I were in our backyard. A beautiful black butterfly landed on a yellow flower blooming in a bush. Charlie looked at me and said, "This is today's gift." I think of that simple statement every day.

Today's gift is there for all of us, if we just open our eyes and unwrap it. It might be a rainbow, an uplifting poem, an unexpected compliment, a smile from a friend, a sunset over the ocean, a candlelit bath, the best ice-cream cone you've ever tasted. There are probably more of these available to you than you realize. It just takes cultivating the habit of looking for them.

Life may throw us off balance, and our resources may run thin, but if we remember to recognize even the smallest of things — those that remind us of how lucky we are to be breathing — then we have found today's gift. These are the moments that when strung together are like the best string of pearls, only better.

Don't let your preparations for tomorrow get in your way of today. Enjoy what happens in your life now, remember what matters, and gather up the gifts in gratitude. They will refresh your soul.

Every single day I want today's gift, that which gives me a sense of delight, appreciation, and love. In the discovery of each day's gifts, I will relish every moment of life and live it to the fullest. And I hope you will, too.

See you at ninety.

RESOURCES

American Cancer Society

1559 Clifton Rd. NE
Atlanta, GA 30329
800-ACS-2345
www.cancer.org
The American Cancer Society (ACS) is a nationwide, community-based voluntary health organization. Headquartered in Atlanta, Georgia, it has state divisions and more than thirty-four hundred local offices. The ACS is dedicated to eliminating cancer as a major health problem by preventing cancer, saving lives, and diminishing suffering from cancer, through research, education, advocacy, and service.

American Diabetes Association

ATTN: National Call Center
1701 North Beauregard St.
Alexandria, VA 22311
800-DIABETES (800-342-2383)

www.diabetes.org
The American Diabetes Association publishes many books and resources for health professionals and people with diabetes, including *Diabetes Forecast,* a monthly magazine for patients, and the journals *Diabetes, Diabetes Care,* and *Diabetes Spectrum.*

American Dietetic Association

120 South Riverside Plaza, Suite 2000
Chicago, IL 60606
800-877-1600
www.eatright.org
The American Dietetic Association is a professional organization that can help you locate a registered dietitian in your community.

American Heart Association

7272 Greenville Ave.
Dallas, TX 75231
800-AHA-USA-1 (800-242-8721)
www.americanheart.org
The American Heart Association is a private, voluntary organization that distributes literature on heart disease and its prevention. Local affiliates can be found in the telephone directory.

American Lung Association

61 Broadway, 6th Floor
New York, NY 10006
212-315-8700
800-LUNGUSA (to contact the American Lung Association nearest you)
www.lungusa.org
The mission of the American Lung Association is to prevent lung disease and promote lung health. Among many other programs, the association offers a variety of smoking control and prevention programs targeted to specific groups — some aimed at adults, others intended for school use, and still others designed to build bridges between the home and school and involve community leaders along with parents and educators.

American Psychological Association

750 First St. NE
Washington, DC 20002
800-374-2721 or 202-336-5500
www.apa.org
The American Psychological Association (APA) is a scientific and professional organization that represents psychology in the United States. The APA's online Psychologist Locator Service can help you find a qualified therapist in your area.

Centers for Disease Control and Prevention

1600 Clifton Rd. NE
Atlanta, GA 30333
Public inquiries: 800-311-3435 or 404-639-3534
www.cdc.gov
The mission of the Centers for Disease Control and Prevention is to promote health and quality of life by preventing and controlling disease, injury, and disability. You'll find current information on vaccinations on its website.

Fertile Hope

65 Broadway, Suite 603
New York, NY 10006
888-994-HOPE or 212-242-6798
www.fertilehope.org
Fertile Hope is a national, nonprofit organization dedicated to providing reproductive information, support, and hope to cancer patients and survivors whose medical treatments present the risk of infertility.

Health Resources and Services Administration

5600 Fishers Ln.
Rockville, MD 20857
www.hrsa.gov

The Health Resources and Services Administration is the primary federal agency for improving access to health-care services for people who are uninsured, isolated, or medically vulnerable.

National Cancer Institute

NCI Public Inquiries Office
6116 Executive Blvd., Room 3036A
Bethesda, MD 20892
800-4-CANCER (800-422-6237)
www.cancer.gov
The National Cancer Institute coordinates the National Cancer Program, which conducts and supports research, training, health information dissemination, and other programs with respect to the cause, diagnosis, prevention, and treatment of cancer; rehabilitation from cancer; and the continuing care of cancer patients and the families of cancer patients.

National Institutes of Health

9000 Rockville Pike
Bethesda, MD 20892
301-496-4000
www.nih.gov
The National Institutes of Health (NIH), a part of the U.S. Department of Health and Human Services, is the primary federal

agency for conducting and supporting medical research. NIH scientists investigate ways to prevent disease as well as the causes, treatments, and even cures for common and rare diseases. Composed of twenty-seven institutes and centers, the NIH provides leadership and financial support to researchers in every state and throughout the world.

National Institute of Mental Health

Science Writing, Press, and Dissemination Branch
6001 Executive Blvd., Room 8184, MSC 9663
Bethesda, MD 20892
866-615-6464 or 301-443-4513
www.nimh.nih.gov
The National Institute of Mental Health is the largest scientific organization in the world dedicated to research focused on the understanding, treatment, and prevention of mental disorders and the promotion of mental health.

National Osteoporosis Foundation

1232 22nd St. NW
Washington, DC 20037
800-231-4222 or 202-223-2226
www.nof.org
To help you locate a doctor to treat your os-

teoporosis, the National Osteoporosis Foundation (NOF) has developed a Professional Partners Network directory. To access this directory, click on "Find a Doctor," then "Find a Doctor Using NOF's Professional Partners Network Directory." Use the pull-down menu for the listing in your state.

National Stroke Association

9707 E. Easter Ln.
Centennial, CO 80112
800-STROKES (800-787-6537)
www.stroke.org
The National Stroke Association makes available to doctors and patients important information and tools for the prevention and treatment of stroke.

Office of Minority Health

Office of the Director
The Tower Building
1101 Wootton Pkwy., Suite 600
Rockville, MD 20852
240-453-2882
www.omhrc.gov
The mission of the Office of Minority Health is to improve and protect the health of racial and ethnic minority populations through the development of health policies and programs that will eliminate health dis-

parities. On its website you'll find many programs that can help the medically denied and the medically vulnerable.

REFERENCES

A portion of the information in this book comes from medical research reports in scientific publications, Internet sources, and computer searches of medical databases of research abstracts.

Myth #1 . . . Annual Checkups Are Obsolete

Nocon, M., et al. 2007. Association of body mass index with heartburn, regurgitation and esophagitis: Results of the Progression of Gastroesophageal Reflux Disease study. *Journal of Gastroenterology and Hepatology* 22:1728–1731.

Prochazka, A. V., et al. 2005. Support of evidence-based guidelines for the annual physical examination: A survey of primary care providers. *Archives of Internal Medicine* 165:2595–2600.

Stefansson, H., et al. 2007. A genetic risk factor for periodic limb movements in sleep. *New England Journal of Medicine* 357:639–647.

Valtin, H. 2003. Drink at least eight glasses of water a day. Really? Is there scientific evidence for "8 × 8"? *American Journal of Physiology* 283:R993–R1004.

Yunsheng, M., et al. 2007. A dietary quality comparison of popular weight-loss plans. *Journal of the American Dietetic Association* 107:1786–1791.

Myth #2 . . . Vaccinations Are Just for Kids

Aiello, A., et al. 2007. Consumer antibacterial soaps: Effective or just risky? *Clinical Infectious Diseases* 45:S137–S147.

Centers for Disease Control and Prevention. 2007. Vaccinations and immunizations, http://www.cdc.gov (accessed September 2007).

Douglas, R. M., et al. 2007. Vitamin C for preventing and treating the common cold. *Cochrane Database of Systematic Reviews* 18:CD000980.

Myth #3 . . . Doctors Don't Play Favorites

American Cancer Society. 2007. Breast cancer facts and figures 2007–2008, http://www.cancer.org (accessed October 2007).

Baker, D. W., et al. 2007. Health literacy and mortality among elderly persons. *Archives of Internal Medicine* 167:1503–1509.

Beal, A. C., et al. 2007. Closing the divide: How medical homes promote equity in health care. Results from The Commonwealth Fund 2006 Health Care Quality Survey. The Commonwealth Fund. June, New York, NY.

Cromie, W. J. 2003. Adding years to your life by reducing your risks. *Harvard Gazette,* August 21. http://www.hno.harvard .edu/gazette/2003/08.21/01-antiaging.html (accessed August 2007).

Flood, J. E., and B. J. Rolls. 2007. Soup preloads in a variety of forms reduce meal energy intake. *Appetite* 49:626–634.

Griggs, J. J., et al. 2007. Effect of patient socioeconomic status and body mass index on the quality of breast cancer adjuvant chemotherapy. *Journal of Clinical Oncology* 25:277–284.

McDaniel, S. H., et al. 2007. Physician self-disclosure in primary care visits — Enough about you, what about me? *Archives of Internal Medicine* 167:1321–1326.

Pogun, S. 2001. Sex differences in brain and behavior: Emphasis on nicotine, nitric oxide and place learning. *International Journal of Psychophysiology* 42:195–208.

Schulman, K. A., et al. 1999. The effect of race and sex on physicians' recommendations for cardiac catheterization. *New England Journal of Medicine* 340:618–626.

Myth #4 . . . Only Old People Get Heart Disease and Stroke

Christakis, N. A., and J. H. Fowler. 2007. The spread of obesity in a large social network over 32 years. *New England Journal of Medicine* 357:370–379.

Dhingra, R., et al. 2007. Soft drink consumption and risk of developing cardiometabolic risk factors and the metabolic syndrome in middle-aged adults in the community. *Circulation* 116:480–488.

Mennella, J. A., et al. 2007. Breastfeeding and smoking: Short-term effects on infant feeding and sleep. *Pediatrics* 120:497–502.

Murray, C. J., et al. 2006. Eight Americas: Investigating mortality disparities across races, counties, and race-counties in the United States. *PLoS Medicine* 3:e260.

Racunica, T. L., et al. 2007. Effect of physical activity on articular knee joint structures in community-based adults. *Arthritis Care & Research* 57:1261–1268.

Salonen, J. T., et al. 1998. Donation of blood is associated with reduced risk of myocardial infarction. The Kuopio Ischaemic Heart Disease Risk Factor Study. *American Journal of Epidemiology* 148:445–451.

University of Maryland Medical Center. 2000. Laughter is good for your heart. News release. November 15, Baltimore, MD.

Myth #5 . . . We're Losing the War on Cancer

Epstein, D. S., et al. 1999. Is physician detection associated with thinner melanomas? *Journal of the American Medical Association* 281:640–643.

Frieden, T. R., and D. E. Blakeman. 2005. The dirty dozen: 12 myths that undermine tobacco control. *American Journal of Public Health* 95:1500–1505.

Garsson, B. 2005. No role for extroversion and neuroticism in cancer development. *Lancet* 366:872–874.

He, X., and R. H. Liu. 2007. Triterpenoids isolated from apple peels have potent antiproliferative activity and may be partially responsible for apple's anticancer activity. *Journal of Agricultural and Food Chemistry* 55:4366–4370.

Hitti, M. 2005, May 16. Statins may cut risk of some cancers, http://www.webmd.com (accessed October 2007).

Kirsh, V. A. 2007. Prospective study of fruit and vegetable intake and risk of prostate cancer. *Journal of the National Cancer Insti-*

tute 99(15):1200–1209.

Larsson, S. C., et al. 2006. Processed meat consumption and stomach cancer risk: A meta-analysis. *Journal of the National Cancer Institute* 98:1078–1087.

McCullough, M. 2003. Calcium, vitamin D, dairy products, and risk of colorectal cancer in the Cancer Prevention Study II Nutrition Cohort (United States). *Cancer Causes and Control* 14:1–12.

Welsh, J. 2007. Vitamin D and prevention of breast cancer. *Acta Pharmacologia Sinica* 28:1373–1382.

Myth #6 . . . *Natural* Means "Safe"

Eden, J. A., et al. 2007. Three cases of endometrial cancer associated with "bioidentical" hormone replacement therapy. *Medical Journal of Australia* 187:244–245.

Hartman, J. W., et al. 2007. Consumption of fat-free fluid milk after resistance exercise promotes greater lean mass accretion than does consumption of soy or carbohydrate in young, novice, male weightlifters. *The American Journal of Clinical Nutrition* 86:373–381.

Izzo, A. A., et al. 2005. Cardiovascular pharmacotherapy and herbal medicines: The risk of drug interaction. *International Journal of Cardiology* 98:1–14.

Izzo, A. A., and E. Ernst. 2001. Interactions between herbal medicines and prescribed drugs: A systematic review. *Drugs* 61:2163–2175.

Kavanaugh, C. J., et al. 2007. The U.S. Food and Drug Administration's evidence-based review for qualified health claims: Tomatoes, lycopene, and cancer. *Journal of the National Cancer Institute* 99:1074–1085.

Kleijnen, J., et al. 1991. Clinical trials of homoeopathy. *British Medical Journal* 302:316–323.

Lawson, K. A., et al. 2007. Multivitamin use and risk of prostate cancer in the National Institutes of Health–AARP Diet and Health Study. *Journal of the National Cancer Institute* 99:754–764.

Lonn, E., et al. 2005. Effects of long-term vitamin E supplementation on cardiovascular events and cancer: A randomized controlled trial. *Journal of the American Medical Association* 293:1338–1347.

Oei, A., and L. R. Hartley. 2005. The effects of caffeine and expectancy on attention and memory. *Human Psychopharmacology* 20:193–202.

Pruthi, S., et al. 2007. Pilot evaluation of flaxseed for the management of hot flashes. *Journal for the Society of Integrative Oncology* 5:106–112.

SanGiovanni, J. P., et al. 2007. The relationship of dietary carotenoid and vitamin A, E, and C intake with age-related macular degeneration in a case-control study: AREDS Report No. 22. *Archives of Ophthalmology* 125:1225–1232.

Shah, S. A., et al. 2007. Evaluation of echinacea for the prevention and treatment of the common cold: A meta-analysis. *Lancet Infectious Diseases* 7:473–480.

Shang, A., et al. 2005. Are the clinical effects of homoeopathy placebo effects? Comparative study of placebo-controlled trials of homoeopathy and allopathy. *Lancet* 366:726–732.

Stranges, S., et al. 2007. Effects of long-term selenium supplementation on the incidence of type 2 diabetes: A randomized trial. *Annals of Internal Medicine* 147:217–223.

Villegas, J. F., et al. 2001. Adverse effects of herbal treatment of cardiovascular disease: What the physician must know. *Heart Disease* 3:169–175.

Vogel, R. A., et al. 2005. ACCF Complementary medicine expert consensus document. *Journal of the American College of Cardiology* 46:184–221.

Von Fraunhofer, J. A., and M. M. Rogers. 2005. Effects of sports drinks and other beverages on dental enamel. *General Dentistry* 53:28–31.

Wahner-Roedler, D. L., et al. 2006. Physicians' attitudes toward complementary and alternative medicine and their knowledge of specific therapies: A survey at an academic medical center. *Evidence-Based Complementary and Alternative Medicine* 3:495–501.

Myth #7 . . . You Can Just Snap Out of Mental Illness

Doheny, K. 2007, August 20. Coping with stress helps cholesterol, http://www.webmd.com (accessed October 2007).

Fiatarone, M., et al. 1994. Exercise training and nutritional supplementation for physical frailty in very elderly people. *New England Journal of Medicine* 330:1769–1775.

Moussavi, S., et al. 2007. Depression, chronic diseases, and decrements in health: Results from the World Health Surveys. *Lancet* 370:851–858.

Pradhan, E. K., et al. 2007. Effect of mindfulness-based stress reduction in rheumatoid arthritis patients. *Arthritis & Rheumatism* 57:1134–1342.

Rush, A. J. 2007. Limitations in efficacy of antidepressant monotherapy. *Journal of*

Clinical Psychiatry 68 (Suppl. 10):8–10.

Shouse, B. 2002. Deadly boring jobs. *Science Now,* May 31. http://sciencenow .sciencemag.org/cgi/content/full/2002/531/ 2 (accessed June 2007).

Zhang, Z., et al. 2007. Blockade of phosphodiesterase Type 5 enhances rat neurohypophysial excitability and electrically evoked oxytocin release. *Journal of Physiology* 584:137–147.

INDEX

Page numbers in *italics* refer to tables.

American Medical Association, 296, 365
amino acids, 278
anaphylaxis, 111
androgens, 294
androstenedione, 278
anemia, 32–33
angina, 335
angiogram, 212
angiotensin-converting enzyme (ACE), 188
angiotensin receptor blockers (ARBs), 188
annual checkups, 25–86, 65
  anxiety about, 81–82
  and changing health, 42–43
  doctor-patient relationship and, 38–43
  family history in, 44
  scheduling, 55, 59
antacids, 32, 298
antibiotics, 105
antibodies, 105
anticonvulsants, 353
antidepressants, 352, 354, 356
antihistamines, 274
antioxidants, 304, 305, 311
antiperspirants, 236
anxiety, 262, 265, 266, 283, 285, 331, 336, 341, 352, 359, 360–361
aortic aneurysm test, 70
aphrodisiacs, 307
apples, 265
aristolochic acid, 278

arnica, 288, 301
arteriosclerosis, 177
arthritis, 20, 52, 159, 231, 272, 335
art therapy, 262
Asclepius, 365–66
ascorbic acid, 109
Asians, 143, 227
aspirin, 203–210, 281
asthma, 18, 335
atherosclerosis, 198, 210, 216
atrial fibrillation (AF), 212–214
Avastin, 258

bacteria, 280
Bauer, Joy, 191
Bechler, Steve, 278
Beck, Jordan, 235
Beck, Lindsay, 222–233, 235–236
Beck, Paisley Jane, 235
bed rest, 154
behavioral therapy, 346
Benadryl, 111
beta-blockers, 188, 214
beta-carotene, 305
bile acid sequestrants, 194
bioidenticals, 294–296
bipolar disorder, 337–341, 339–342, 353
birth control pills, 281
bitter orange, 279, 282
blindness, prevented by sunglasses, 82

cancer (*continued*)

cholesterol (*continued*)
  coffee and, 191
  drugs for, 18
  in eggs, 186
  HDL, 195, 334
  heart disease and, 181, 196
  LDL, 61, 191, 194–195, 204
  screening for, 37, *65*
chondroitin, 279
chronotherapy, 17–18
clot, 212
COBRA, 139
coenzyme Q-10, 279
coffee, 47, 191, 283, 315
cognitive therapy, 346
colds, 17, 103, 107, 109
collagen-to-mineral ratio, 30
colon:
  aspirin and, 203
  cancer of, 27–28, 32, 38, 63, 143, 171, 231, 239, 245–257, 265–268, 284, 293
  cleansing of, 284
  smoking and, 128
colonoscopies, 26–28, 63, *68*
colorectal health, *67*
comfrey, 278
community health center locator, 130
complementary treatments, 273, 312–315
  for cancer, 261–268
computed tomography (CT), 34–35,

fats, 204
  monounsaturated, 196, 204
  saturated, 171, 195, 239, 370
  trans, 171, 196, 370
fennel seeds, 287
feverfew, 286
fevers, 19, 115
fiber, 195, 239, 279
fibric acids, 194
fibrocystic breasts, 283
fight/flight reflex, 332
fish oil, 204
flaxseed, 296
folic acid, 178
Food and Drug Administration, U.S., 36, 103, 119, 207, 236, 277, 278, 294, 309
free radicals, 195
fruits, 47, 171, 195, 219, 303, 348, 370, 379

gallbladder disease, 135
garcinia cambogia, 282
garlic, 287
gastroesophageal reflux disease (GERD), 61
gastrointestinal problems, 283
genes, 44–45, 143, 253
  acne and, 151
  earwax and, 227
  heart attacks and, 195

heart disease (*continued*)
  homeopathy and, 300
  inactivity and, 154
  iron and, 195
  obesity and, 170
  Ornish diet for, 54
  race and, 138–139
  risk factors for, 181, 196
  smoking and, 200
  soft drinks and, 184
  vegetables and, 171
Helicobacter, 100
Hendrix, Leean, 178–179
hepatitis A, 116, 117
hepatitis B, 118
hepatitis C, 118
HER-2 receptor, 256
herbal medicine, 261, 281–287, 287–288,
  289–290, 300, 307
herbs, 275
heroin, 242
herpes, 99
heterocyclicamines (HCAs), 264
hiccups, 313
high blood sugar, 35
high-risk pools, 140
Hippocrates, 275–276
Hispanics, 139, 143
histamine, 113
HIV, 98, 173

positron emission tomography (PET), 240, 259

postpartum depression, 326

potassium, 199

poverty, 143

Pravachol, 252

prayer, 262

pregnancy, 304

pregnancy care, 133

premenstrual syndrome, 283

prenatal tests, 82

progesterone, 294

proteins, 122, 186

Prozac, 353, 357

PSA tests, 60

psychodynamic therapy, 346

psychoneuroimmunology (PNI), 265

radiation, 256

radio frequency ablation, 256

radiologists, 60

raspberry tea, 287

rectal exam, *68*

rectum, cancer of, 247, 293

relaxation therapy, 261

remission, 259

Requip, 84

restless leg syndrome (RLS), 84

retinol, 286

Reye's syndrome, 209

smoking (*continued*)
  women and, 174
snakeroot, 278
sneezing, 182
soaps, 107
sodium, 170
soup, 170
soy, 113
sperm, 147
spina bifida, 179
spinach, 303
spine, CT and, 34
spiral CT, 253
spirituality, 262
staph infections, 107
statins, 194
steroids, 32
stinging nettles, 287
stomach flu, 117
stress, 43, 55, 246, 262, 266, 329, 332,
  349, 370, 372
  cholesterol and, 334
  exercise and, 248
  gray hair and, 361
  heart disease and, 180
  pets and, 321
  shingles and, 88
  ulcers and, 101
stress test, 49
strokes, 22, 183

tobacco, 269
tocopherols, 302
tocotrienols, 302
tomatoes, 293
toothbrushes, 92
trans fats, 171, 196, 370
transient ischemic attack (TIA), 215
triage, 128
triglycerides, 192, 197
troches, 294
T-scores, 29
tumors, 123, 237, 248, 250, 255, 258

ulcerative colitis, 324
ulcers, 61, 100, 136, 210, 283
ultrasound, 49, 156, 211, 252
urinalysis, 37
UVA rays, 249
UVB rays, 249

vaccines, 105, 296–299
  for cancer, 123
  for DTP, 108
  for flu, 117
  for hepatitis, 118
  for HPV, 104, 110
  for measles, 97, 98
  for measles, mumps, and rubella, 112
  for meningococcal meningitis, 92, 104, 119

ABOUT THE AUTHOR

Nancy L. Snyderman, M.D., F.A.C.S., is the chief medical editor for NBC News and reports for *Nightly News* with Brian Williams, *Today,* and MSNBC. She also has an academic appointment in the Department of Otolaryngology–Head and Neck Surgery at the University of Pennsylvania. Prior to joining NBC News, Dr. Snyderman served as a medical correspondent for ABC News, then spearheaded a digital project at Johnson & Johnson. She has received numerous broadcasting awards and grants from the American Cancer Society and the Kellogg Foundation. Dr. Snyderman lives on the East Coast with her family. She is passionate about horses, travel, and hiking.

The employees of Thorndike Press hope you have enjoyed this Large Print book. All our Thorndike, Wheeler, and Kennebec Large Print titles are designed for easy reading, and all our books are made to last. Other Thorndike Press Large Print books are available at your library, through selected bookstores, or directly from us.

For information about titles, please call:
(800) 223-1244

or visit our Web site at:
http://gale.cengage.com/thorndike

To share your comments, please write:
Publisher
Thorndike Press
295 Kennedy Memorial Drive
Waterville, ME 04901